ETHICS IN ACTION

BIOMEDICAL ETHICS

CONCEPTS AND CASES FOR HEALTH CARE PROFESSIONALS

SAUL ROSS, Ed.D.
University of Ottawa

DAVID CRUISE MALLOY, Ph.D.
University of Regina

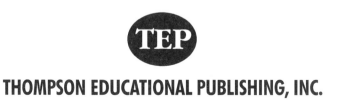

THOMPSON EDUCATIONAL PUBLISHING, INC.

Requests for permission to make copies of any part of the work should be directed to the publisher: www.thompsonbooks.com.

Copies of this book may be ordered in the United States and Canada from our distributor:

United States:
General Distribution Services Limited
85 River Rock Drive, #202
Buffalo, New York 14207
Toll Free: 1-800-805-1083
Fax: (416) 213-1917

Canada:
General Distribution Services Limited
325 Humber College Boulevard
Toronto, Ontario M9W 7C3
1-800-387-0141 (ON/QC)
1-800-387-0172 (rest of Canada)
Fax: (416) 213-1917

email: customer.service@ccmailgw.genpub.com

Cataloguing in Publication Data

Ross, Saul, 1934-
   Biomedical ethics : concepts and cases for health care professionals

Includes bibliographical references.
ISBN 1-55077-090-X

1. Bioethics. 2. Bioethics - Case studies. I. Malloy, David Cruise, 1959-
II. Title.

QH332.R67 1999   174'.25   C98-932641-1

Copyediting by: Elizabeth Phinney.
Cover illustration: Leon Zernitsky.
Cover design: Elan Designs.

We acknowledge the support of the Government of Canada through the Book Publishing Industry Development Program for our publishing activities.
Printed in Canada.
1 2 3 4 5   06 05 04 03 02 01 00 99

Table of Contents

Case Studies

Acknowledgments

In any venture such as this, assistance from a number of sources is obtained. Our gratitude is hereby expressed to the following people who were so generous with their time, knowledge and advice: Angela Kramer, Dr. S. Kardash, Dr. M. Richter, Dr. R. Rivington, Dr. R. Saginur and Dr. V. Sistek. Special thanks go to the late Dr. L. Charette.

We dedicate this text to some very important people in our lives who provide us with constant inspiration and courage:

- To Saul's wife, Pamela Ross, to their daughters and husbands, Karyn and Brian, Dana and John, and to their grandchildren, Quinton and Serena; and
- To David's wife, Valerie Loy Sluth, and their children Connor, Gaelan and Bronwen.

Preface

Rarely does a week pass without the media reporting on some ethical controversy related to health care. This attention has served both to educate the public and alert it to what transpires in hospitals, medical laboratories, clinics, practitioners' offices, nursing homes, rehabilitation settings and even in medical and nursing schools. Nevertheless, while the public has some interest in these matters, it is health care practitioners who have a greater concern since their profession and their livelihood is directly involved.

Recent scientific and technological advances have propelled a great number of biomedical topics to the forefront, matters which present themselves as perplexing, and at times confounding, ethical dilemmas. Abortion, the right to refuse treatment, informed consent, a change in the physician-patient relationship, euthanasia, DNR, human experimentation, allocation of scarce resources and reproductive technology—these do not nearly exhaust the list of topics, yet each is fraught with ethical issues.

During the past three or four decades, a sizable literature has emerged on these and other biomedical ethical issues. Unfortunately, much of this literature is abstract and theoretical, making it too remote for health care students (and perhaps even philosophers). Much of the rest focuses on how one ought to behave in practical settings without regard to moral reasoning at all. The remainder of the literature tries to bridge the gap between theory and practice by analyzing cases within the context of either the various principles or established ethical theories.

While there is value in these approaches, there is one major drawback—the readers do not themselves engage in moral discourse, but rather it is handed down to them. Since the analysis is done for them, they are, in effect, deprived of the opportunity to hone their own analytical skills; they do not participate actively in moral reasoning. As all educators know, there is a difference between learning by observing others (in these situations, reading the sage comments of the authors) and learning by doing. This volume seeks to redress this shortcoming, so that students can learn to grapple with issues as they may arise.

Medicine comprises a technical and an ethical component which are indissoluble. It is common practice for all graduating medical students to swear an oath prior to practice—be it the Hippocratic oath, the Oath According to

Hippocrates In So Far As a Christian May Swear It or the (Hebrew) Physician's Oath of Asaph. Whichever oath is sworn matters little, as each imposes certain responsibilities on physicians, both technical and ethical, for as long as they practice medicine. Health care professionals are carefully educated to ensure the highest level of proficiency on the technical side. Since there is an ethical component in all medical practice, we believe that the same educational approach should be used for this component; namely exposure to theory and ample opportunity to practice. Prudent health care practice requires expertise in two realms: profound knowledge of the biophysical sciences and the technical practices rooted therein, and knowledge of ethics, along with the analytical skills needed to apply that knowledge. Good human relations skills, based on knowledge gleaned from the psychosocial sciences, add another valuable dimension, which will enable the health care professional to practice in a more comprehensive manner.

Guided by the belief that health care practitioners need both a base in ethics as well as ample opportunities to engage in moral discourse, this book will

- introduce a number of basic concepts in ethics;
- provide models which will serve to guide moral discourse (These models need not be followed rigidly; they are designed to orient the discussion so that it flows in a comprehensive and orderly fashion.);
- identify a number of basic medical principles along with various conceptions of medical practice to serve as the context for moral discourse; and
- provide case material, based on actual events, that will allow students an opportunity to engage in moral discourse.

We hope to effect a somewhat better balance between the theoretical and practical. Above all, we are convinced that this method will enable health care practitioners to make more intelligent decisions when they are faced with moral dilemmas.

1

Introduction

New Approaches to Medical Education

It is not so long ago that students in the various health care schools spent almost all of their time in classrooms and laboratories. As time progressed changes were made to place more emphasis on practice in an attempt to improve the blend between the theoretical and practical components. What transpired in medical schools serves as an example to illustrate the changes made to the flow of the educational experience.

Although medicine is considered an undergraduate program, the vast majority of students admitted already possess an undergraduate degree, most often specializing in one of the basic sciences, such as biology or chemistry. During the four-year medical school program, it was not unusual to find that the entire first three years were consigned to the basic sciences; this block was usually referred to as the pre-clinical years or the pre-clinical component of the curriculum. Courses in the biophysical sciences, for example, anatomy and physiology, were structured to provide students with extensive and comprehensive knowledge of human biological structures, as well as knowledge of the circulatory, respiratory, digestive and nervous systems.

To further enhance this body of theory, additional courses were offered in histology, neuroanatomy, pharmacology, physics, chemistry and biochemistry. Insights and understandings about how the body functions at the micro and macro levels were thereby gleaned. An advanced level of scientific knowledge, including an in-depth mastery of the wide array of knowledge presented, was the goal sought. In such programs, it was not until the fourth year, when clerkship was first scheduled, that medical students began to see patients in hospital.

Diagnostic skills and therapeutic regimes were then learned in the traditional, time-honored fashion of doing rounds with residents and staff physicians. As cases were presented, clerks and interns were called upon to assess each situation and, in so doing, began to acquire and improve the requisite abilities. There may have been some consideration given to ethical aspects during these discussions but, due to the invariable pressure of time and the large number of cases scheduled for review, it is safe to assume that the major

focus of attention was on acquiring diagnostic skills and, as a logical extension, learning what and how to prescribe, thereby enhancing the students'
knowledge of the practice of medicine.

The basic assumption underlying this approach to medical education can
be summarized as follows: a comprehensive, in-depth body of theory is a
prerequisite for understanding illness and the steps that need to be taken to
restore health. However, medical theory, by itself, is insufficient to help those
who are ill; diagnostic skills and the prescription of therapeutic measures are
required in order to help the patient get better. Although it appears redundant,
to complete the picture, it is equally valid to state that diagnosing and prescribing ring hollow without a solid base of scientific theory. In order to
practice medicine a physician needs theoretical knowledge and therapeutic
skills. (Another component will be proposed shortly.)

Jonsen and Toulmin (1988) aptly describe the situation:

> Medicine blends theory and practice, intellectual grasp and technical skill,
> *episteme* and *phronesis*, in its own characteristic manner. It spans the spec-
> trum of Theory and Practice, from the general theories of biomedical sci-
> ence at one extreme to the particular procedures of clinical practice at the
> other. In doing so it illustrates the complex and subtle ways in which theo-
> retical and practical knowledge bear on each other. At one extreme, medi-
> cine overlaps into the natural sciences. Research in physiology and other
> biomedical fields aims to refine our general ideas (specifically, our general
> ideas about health and disease) quite as much as research in any other
> science. The central core of medicine, however, comprises practical proce-
> dures designed not to explain health and disease in theory but to treat illness
> and restore health, as a matter of practice (p.41).

Both components, theory and practice, need to be acquired by the physician in
order to practice medicine. What has been questioned is the order in which
theory and practice, technical knowledge and skilled intervention, is to be
learned, as well as how to blend them. What has changed in the medical
school curriculum is when the practical aspect, clerkship, has been introduced
as well as the amount of time allocated to that component.

By far the most radical change in formulating the medical school curriculum occurred at McMaster University's School of Medicine (located in Ham-
ilton, Ontario, Canada) three decades ago. The curriculum was completely
revamped. Theory and practice were blended right from the outset. In contrast
to other medical schools where the study of theory (basic sciences) came first,
it seemed that at McMaster practice either came first or was allotted equal
time with theory. Students, working in small groups and using a problem-
solving approach, were introduced to patients (the first few were actors por-
traying patients) at the beginning of their education. Shortly thereafter,
clerkship began and students spent time in physicians' offices and in hospitals

observing diagnoses and treatments. Changes also came about in medical schools with traditional curricula; students no longer needed to wait until their fourth year for clerkship experience, but could begin as early as the second year.

Much of the discussion about the ideal sequence and blend of theory and practice is often framed in terms of when clerkship ought to begin and how large a portion of the curriculum it should command. In these debates the question of what constitutes an adequate theoretical base emerges. Without sufficient theory, it is argued, students will not profit from their presence in a clinical setting. What is rarely mentioned in this context is the ethical component of medical practice, nor is there much time set aside in the curriculum in Canadian universities for that topic (Baylis and Downie, 1990).

Insufficient attention paid to the ethical component of medical practice in the curriculum may mean that the educational preparation of physicians is incomplete. This gap shows up early, when students enter the clinical environment. Loewy (1987) brings this issue to light in a clear and forceful manner.

> When physicians in training enter the clinical years and first begin to become involved in clinical decision making, they soon find that more than the technical data they had so carefully learned is involved. Prior to that time, of course, they were aware that more than technology was involved in practicing medicine, but here, for the first time, the reality is forcefully brought home. It may be on a medical ward, when a patient or a patient's relatives ask that no further treatment be given and that the patient be allowed to die; it may be in ob/gyn, when a 4- or 5-month pregnant lady with two other children and just deserted by her husband pleads for an abortion; it may be in the outpatient setting, where patients unable to afford enough to eat cannot afford to buy antibiotics for their sick child or provide him or her with the recommended diet (p.ix).

Advice on how to address these, and a host of similar ethical dilemmas which will confront all practitioners, cannot be sought from the body of scientific theory, nor will assistance be provided in diagnostic skills and therapeutic procedures. Difficult choices need to be made and there is a source, ethics, which may be of help.

Many changes have occurred in medical education, particularly with regard to blending theory and practice, and these initiatives represent new approaches to medical education. However, as Baylis and Downie (1990) report, very little time is allocated to ethics, and within the time allotted, questions must be raised about the exposure to theory and the opportunities afforded students to practice applied ethics.

Parallel Approaches to the Ethical Component

Medical practice, and by extension all health care practice, can be described as consisting of two component parts: technical, where scientific theory and practice are inextricably combined, and ethical. As noted in the preceding section, the medical school curriculum has undergone significant changes on the technical side with regard to the blending of theory and practice. Ethics, as a specific subject area, is a relative newcomer to the curriculum. Not only is its place and time allocation still open to debate but there appears to be some disagreement about what is to be taught and how the material is to be covered. For example, Baylis and Downie (1990) question whether or not ethical theory should be included at all in medical ethics courses.

Careful consideration needs to be given to both the content of and pedagogical procedures used in medical ethics courses. A stern caveat has been issued by Veatch (1977): "Physicians must no longer be educated as technical geniuses and moral imbeciles" (p.v). That pronouncement may be too harsh as a blanket indictment, yet it appears to have some import in serving as a directive to ensure that medical ethics courses are of the highest quality and achieve their stated objectives.

Medical students, like everyone else in society, have some general knowledge of ethics and behave in a moral fashion. From infancy, they have been taught by others, such as parents, relatives, teachers, camp counselors and religious officials, how to behave properly. This normative "education" generally produces law-abiding, considerate, well-behaved, moral individuals, but it does not provide them with a theoretical base to explain why some acts are right while others are wrong, why some behavior is good but other behavior is bad, and why some conduct is authentic, yet other conduct is inauthentic (*authentic* and *inauthentic* are terms applied to situations where an individual critically examines his or her own behavior).

Courses in medical ethics need to go beyond what students have learned about proper conduct from parents and other persons of influence. With regard to both content and pedagogy, there are certain parallels which can be drawn between the technical component of the curriculum and the ethical component.

> The learning and practice of medical ethics in a clinical setting requires many of the same structures and dynamics as the learning and practice of medicine. Practical ethical training must also, like clinical medicine, be preceded by extensive study of ethical principles, structures and systems (Ellos, 1990, p.2).

A blend of both the theoretical and the practical, that is, applied ethics, is required. Theory cannot be omitted and applied ethics must be learned, because moral dilemmas will emerge constantly in practice.

Teaching students moral theory in medical ethics courses is an objective rarely mentioned by the respondents to the survey of Canadian medical schools conducted by Baylis and Downie (1990, p.31). Students need: some guidance on how to recognize ethical issues and dilemmas; to become familiar with the ethical principles that guide much of medical practice; opportunities to delve into the meaning of the various oaths and codes of behavior which apply to medical practice; to be made aware of community mores, particularly now that almost all of us live in multicultural communities; and instruction in how to develop analytical skills which will enhance ethical decision making. However, as Ellos (1990) has pointed out, they also need to study ethical theory and have ample practice in doing applied ethics.

Just as theory and practice in the technical component of medicine are combined in clinical practice so, too, must ethical theory and its application be present. Comprehension of ethical theory extends the students' horizons and deepens their understanding of the dilemma at hand, beyond what they have learned about their own proper comportment. Practice in doing applied ethics provides the students with opportunities to sharpen their analytical skills, thus helping them to develop greater insights into problematic situations. By engaging in moral discourse, they are encouraged to state reasons for their observations and viewpoints and, by so doing, they come to appreciate the intellectual demands of this line of thinking.

Where ethical theory is not included, questions must be raised about how effective medical education courses can be in achieving their objectives. Without a foundation in ethical theory to serve as an intellectual base, discussion is much more likely to fall into the realm of opinion. Since each of us is entitled to our own opinion, not much, if any, intellectual advancement will be made if the discussion remains at that level.

Studying ethical theory as an end in itself is a worthwhile academic endeavor, one containing a myriad of fascinating challenges. This, by and large, is the domain of philosophy. While medical students might come to appreciate the lure of philosophy, their immediate concern, and justifiably so, centers on the relevance and applicability of ethics to medicine. More specifically, their interest is in the applied aspect, in acquiring intellectual tools to help them address actual complex moral situations. Just as they rely on their knowledge of anatomy, physiology, chemistry and pharmacology to help them treat patients so, too, should they look to their knowledge of ethical theory to enable them to address moral dilemmas. Both components of medical practice are rooted in theory.

Both theory and practice are addressed within this text. Our approach differs from what is found in other books, where the emphasis is placed either on the theoretical side (exposition of some ethical theories and/or discussion of the various ethical principles which apply to medical practice) or attempts are made to blend the two. In the latter case, the authors engage in moral discourse by doing the ethical analysis for the readers. In this text, we expound a number of ethical theories and discuss the pertinent principles that apply to medicine, present two models to guide moral discourse so that analytic skills can be developed through practice, and provide many cases for analysis. It is the reader, not the authors, who will do the analysis. They will engage in moral discourse that is rooted in theory and guided by models to help them attain comprehensiveness and progress in a logical fashion.

On the technical side, students now learn diagnostic and therapeutic skills much earlier by actually engaging in practice. On the ethical side, and in a parallel fashion, we are convinced that they should also have the opportunity to acquire the analytical skills needed to engage in moral discourse by doing. That goal will be accomplished by addressing the cases presented in the book.

A Brief Overview of Content and Approach Used

Based on the material presented in the first two sections of Chapter 1, it is clear that one of our goals is to blend ethical theory and applied ethics. Furthermore, through the study of the cases presented in the last chapter, ample opportunity exists for the readers to actually do applied ethics. To make that exercise meaningful and fruitful from an educational perspective, familiarity with some ethical theories is needed to serve as an intellectual foundation. Two models, one basic and the other more complex, are offered to help guide moral discourse and ethical decision making. Taken together, these components serve as a framework within which moral reasoning is conducted.

There is a logical flow to the order in which the material is introduced. Reference has already been made to the presence of an ethical component in all biomedical situations. In Chapter 2, some of the technological innovations that have emerged recently are examined, and some of the new conceptualizations that have appeared, particularly with regard to the cessation of life, will be discussed. Attention is directed toward showing how these advances have not only highlighted certain ethical dilemmas but, at the same time, have created new and more difficult moral problems. Anyone currently practicing medicine must be well versed in ethics in order to deal with these complex, and at times heart-wrenching, issues.

The first steps in establishing a theoretical foundation are taken in Chapter 3. Basic concepts in ethics are introduced, along with a number of definitions to help ensure a common understanding of the terms used. Three ethical theories are described very briefly in preparation for a more detailed discussion in the following chapter. An important feature is the emphasis placed on identifying and enunciating an ethical maxim that will serve as a yardstick against which behavior can be measured.

A basic, five-step model is presented as a guide for moral discourse. This is a suggested procedure, one which need not be followed in a lock-step fashion, but which can be used to achieve a comprehensive discussion of the issue at hand. Utilization of this model facilitates the applied components of ethics since its goal is to help the user render moral judgment.

Chapter 4 contains a more detailed account of three ethical theories: consequentialism (teleology), non-consequentialism (deontology), and existentialism. As the explication evolves, the strengths and weaknesses, the advantages and disadvantages as well as the limitations of each theory are discussed. Through this exploration the notions of good, right and authentic become a little clearer.

Behavior is the overt manifestation of decisions made by the agent. To improve our understanding of appropriate behavior, there is a need to examine various factors that influence the decision-making process. These factors or moderators are the focus of Chapter 5; their study provides deeper insight into what prompts people to act in certain ways. Reference to these moderators, during moral discourse, sheds additional light on the issues and may influence the final pronouncement.

A second, more sophisticated, model is included here, one which is designed to guide ethical decision making during deliberations prior to acting. It can also be applied to help the user render moral judgments. This model takes into account aspects of individual moral development as well as psychological and social moderators. Its more comprehensive structure serves to remind those engaged in moral discourse or in making decisions to account for many more factors.

Emanating from Chapter 5, but geared toward facilitating the practical side, is a seven-step process to guide ethical decision making presented in Chapter 6. Its applicability will be obvious to anyone faced with a true-life ethical dilemma; its usefulness will be seen when the cases presented in Chapter 9 are studied.

In Chapter 7, five basic ethical principles which guide medical practice are identified: nonmaleficence, beneficence, confidentiality, respect for individual autonomy and justice. Each is briefly expounded upon to provide the specific context for the analysis of the cases. To serve as additional context, a number of models of medical practice are also listed, since each has its own set of values in caring for patients and a vision of how medicine should function. These principles and models could influence the moral judgment rendered in each case.

Chapter 8 contains trial runs with two models in order to give the reader a general idea of how one might approach the cases that follow in the final chapter. Here, one case is analyzed, guided by the models presented and discussed within the context of the special considerations noted in the preceding chapter. This analysis is meant as a demonstration of how to proceed.

A wide range of cases are presented in Chapter 9. Now, armed with basic concepts in ethics, an understanding of three ethical theories, an appreciation for the use of an ethical maxim, and assisted by models which guide moral discourse, ample opportunities are available in the form of actual cases to engage in moral discourse.

Two well-known pedagogical principles—start at the level of the learner and from there advance to more complex material, and learn by doing—have guided the approach used in this book. Based on the assumption that some readers have limited background in the study of ethics, basic concepts have been introduced first. That step has been followed by an exposition of three ethical theories which serve as a conceptual foundation for the applied aspect. Two models to guide moral discourse and ethical decision making have then been advanced to facilitate the blending of theory and practice.

Learning by doing is implemented in this final chapter, where the case studies are presented. As each case is examined and analyzed, the reader will learn by doing. Since the cases cover a wide range of issues, many aspects of biomedical practice are explored as the reader practices his or her analytical skills during moral discourse. Wrestling with these cases will make the reader morally sensitive. Exploration of these moral dilemmas should provide future practitioners with some basis for addressing the difficult situations they will meet once they start practicing in the field of medicine.

Advice on How to Use This Book

There is some reluctance on our part to offer pedagogical advice, since each professor has his or her own favorite teaching methods as well as ideas on how best to proceed. That reluctance is tempered by the awareness that even the most experienced teachers can benefit from the suggestions offered by colleagues who have tried something different. Adopting new approaches is readily justified if the method used facilitates learning.

A review of the table of contents and the elaboration presented in the preceding section would, at first glance, seem to indicate how to proceed: master the basic concepts, learn the theories, study the models, discuss the special medical ethical principles and the models of medical practice which constitute the specific context and then institute small discussion groups to address the case studies. That certainly is one way to proceed, but a word of caution might be in order; students may become restless if they are confined to the realm of theory for too long. Alternative approaches are available, procedures which will retain the blending of theory and practice and maintain the interest of students.

One possibility is to start the course with a case study. As the discussion evolves, the instructor is in a position to question some of the comments made. These queries, formulated properly, will expose some of the lacunae due to the lack of knowledge of ethical theories. Lack of knowledge of ethical theory limits the scope and progress of the discussion. When such an intervention is successful, the need to study ethical theories becomes obvious to everyone.

As successful as that procedure may be, it does not necessarily mean that all the theoretical material must be completed before any other cases are addressed. It is pedagogically possible, indeed feasible, to intersperse the study of theoretical material with the applied component in small group discussions.

Another interesting approach can be attempted if there is sufficient time available. Very early in the course, before the theoretical aspects are studied, the discussion of a few cases can be recorded. After some aspects of theory have been addressed, the same cases can be revisited to determine if the discussion is now on a higher level and if more penetrating comments are being made which lead to new insights. Once again the theoretical and the practical can be blended in a different way.

As each case is studied, the identification of an ethical maxim will serve as a yardstick against which behavior is measured. Much educational benefit can be derived by promoting discussion of this challenging task. At times, difficulties may be encountered in enunciating a maxim, and at other times, consensus may not be reached regarding which specific maxim is directly applicable. When various suggestions are offered, it indicates that the moral issue is defined or conceptualized in a different way by different members of the group. Much can be learned about ethics from these debates.

Case studies, as a useful pedagogical procedure, are used in many academic settings. Each case provides a common base for discussion and, through participation in small groups, allows everyone to become actively involved. Through the give-and-take that ensues, new insights emerge as the discussion evolves. However, there are some potential problems with small group discussions. Irrelevant material can be introduced, the group can become mired in dealing with minor points and the discussion can become too narrowly focused or too broadly diffused. There may be times when all theoretical aspects are omitted as very "practical" solutions are sought. Although there are no assurances, it is anticipated that the judicious application of the models designed to guide moral discourse found in this text will serve to direct the discussion along the most fruitful path and keep the deliberation focused on the key issues.

2

It's a Different World

Pretend for a moment that the year is 1950, the mid-point of the twentieth century, and that we have the ability to peer into the functioning of a large, well-equipped hospital staffed by highly qualified physicians, surgeons, nurses, technologists and therapists. Suppose we could list all the machines, technical instruments and procedures used to assist in diagnosis and treatment and enumerate the medication available for prescription to help cure the range of illness identified. Suppose, à la Rip Van Winkle, we could anaesthetize all the health care professionals and wake them up some fifty years later situated in a contemporary modern hospital with all the newest equipment, medication and diagnostic and therapeutic procedures. Astonishment, at the very least, would likely be their collective reaction. While some aspects of health care would be the same, such as the importance of the physician-patient relationship and the need for a thorough patient history, much else would be radically different.

Medical Practice, Research and Ethics

Research and technology in the past half-century has enabled the medical community to transplant organs. "Clinical organ transplantation started in 1954 with the first successful kidney transplant which was carried out at the Peter Bent Brigham Hospital by Dr. Joseph Murray" (Sells, 1990, p.1003). That event appears to have motivated other physicians, such as Dr. Christian Barnard, whose first efforts to transplant human hearts captured worldwide interest and served to expand medical horizons even farther. New procedures were invented; renal patients are kept alive and functioning through dialysis. Very premature infants, who fifty years ago had no chance of surviving, are kept alive in neonatal intensive care units. Through the use of amniocentesis and ultrasound examinations, abnormalities in the fetus can be detected and, at times, surgery can be performed to correct what is malfunctioning while the fetus is still in the womb.

Fibre optics changed medical practice radically in certain specialties. A variety of scopes, introduced into bodily orifices, project clear pictures of various organs and other body parts on the monitor to facilitate both diagnosis and surgery. Pharmaceutical companies develop new, and often much more expensive, medication. Companies which manufacture medical equipment are continuously inventing new products, for example, the MRI machine, which can do much more than X-ray equipment. Costs for health care, as a percentage of the Gross National Product (GNP) of each Western industrialized country, have risen dramatically.

Telemetry allows one health care professional to monitor a variety of signs in many patients at the same time. Indeed the equipment is so sophisticated that special sounds alert the staff when any deviation occurs. Respirators keep patients, who are unable to breathe on their own, alive. Life can be prolonged almost indefinitely, or until such time as consent is given to shut off the respirator so that the patient can die with dignity. Other scenarios can be sketched. Respirators can prolong the life of a patient until consent is given to harvest the organs for the purpose of transplanting them in critically ill patients on waiting lists.

Major scientific and technological changes have emerged in the past half-century. Focusing on the beginning of life, we have witnessed dramatic changes in conception (in vitro fertilization, surrogate motherhood), prenatal diagnosis, genetic screening and counseling, and fetal therapy, to highlight but a few. Focusing on the end of life, changes have occurred in the way we care for the dying and how we think about the termination of treatment, including attempts to draw distinctions between ordinary and extraordinary care, and careful consideration has been given to distinguishing between acts of omission and acts of commission in the care of the dying. As will be discussed shortly, the notion of death has been reconceptualized.

Major advances in medicine are not confined to only the beginning and end of life; all aspects of health care have been affected. We have witnessed "what some have called a biomedical revolution" (Harron, Burnside and Beauchamp, 1983, p.xi). Our goal here is not to focus on technology but rather to examine the consequences of these scientific changes which have, in effect, altered reality. Harron et al. (1983) offer a pertinent comment:

> In the past, the physician and other health care professionals have stood by in relative helplessness in the face of many diseases; now the health care profession manages a technological arsenal. For the treatment of many illnesses and injuries new options are available, which, even when they cannot produce recovery, may greatly affect the circumstances of life and death (p.xi).

Certain consequences, most often ethical in nature, flow therefrom.

Advances in science and technology have enabled health care professionals to affect the circumstances of life and death. These new practices and conceptions raise serious questions about the nature of disease (including what constitutes a disease), allocation of resources (e.g., how long to keep a patient on a respirator), the propriety of genetic intervention, what constitutes life and what constitutes death (Kluge, 1992, p.xii). Rapid technological advances have given rise to a great number of new and difficult ethical problems. Perhaps the most fundamental issue raised is the very notion of personhood.

Two seemingly similar, but actually widely divergent, questions can be posed: What is a person?; and Who is a person? Implicit in the first question is the view of a person as an object, a thing which can be weighed and measured, poked and prodded, and kept breathing through the use of machines. Subjectivity may, or may not, be an attribute when persons are considered solely as objects. In sharp contrast the latter query, Who is a person?, attributes subjectivity to that being. That being, as a subject, has rights and bears responsibility for his or her intentional actions. Since the "focus in all biomedical ethics is the person" (Francoeur, 1983, p.183), there is a need to determine who qualifies as a person.

On what basis do we determine who qualifies as a person? While this may be a question which cannot be answered fully, attempts must be made to arrive at an operational definition. How the former question, Who is a person?, is answered has profound ethical implications as well as serious consequences for medical practice, particularly with reference to the beginnings of life and the cessation of life. Scientific developments and advances in medical technology have complicated the issue, making the task of answering this fundamental question even more of a challenge.

A somewhat analogous manner of raising the issue, one which emerges clearly in medical practice is to discuss the differences between the sanctity of life compared to the quality of life (Callahan, 1990). Framing the topic in this manner directs our attention to the end of life and what, if anything, should be done from a medical perspective. *Sanctity of life* is a concept with deep historic roots. Life is to be preserved whenever possible, for as long as possible, and treatment should be undertaken and maintained to achieve that goal. *Quality of life* is a term which subtly instructs the physician to take into account many other factors; preservation of life, under any and all circumstances, is no longer the chief value.

These issues, ethical in nature, merit serious consideration since they will arise in practice on an ongoing basis.

Prior to addressing these issues directly another aspect relating to the technological revolution merits a brief comment. Amongst the wide array of programs broadcast by the television networks are a number of shows that either revolve around the practice of medicine or are set in a hospital. At times the emergency room is the setting while at other times it is the operating theatre. One network telecasts actual surgery being performed. Invariably viewers see patients connected to, and monitored by, the latest sophisticated technology which is often controlled by computers. By the time the program ends severely ill "patients" have been cured, or saved, or are well on the way to recovery. Viewers, far removed from the actual practice of medicine, have been "educated" about modern medical technology. When they become ill they could well have unrealistically high levels of expectation since they have seen so many miracle cures on television. From an ethical perspective, health care professionals, at all levels of care, may find it beneficial for everyone involved to raise this matter when discussing treatment options with their patients.

Technological Innovations, New Conceptualizations and Ethics

Issues before Birth

It is not so long ago that the range of treatments available to the medical community to treat infertility was severely limited. After other possible impediments were ruled out, the obstetrician examining an infertile woman focused on her fallopian tubes to determine if they were the source of the problem. If the diagnosis confirmed the suspicion, and surgical intervention could not correct the situation, the attending physician had few, if any, other options available to help the patient achieve a pregnancy. With the natural means of procreation unavailable, adoption was often the alternative recommended.

Inability to conceive, whether due to problems of subfertility or infertility, impinges on a deep-felt need; many couples afflicted with this problem experience pain and anguish. Social and psychological pressure, at times very subtle, at other times overt, is exerted on childless couples. Even the quality of the couple's relationship can be adversely affected if they are unable to conceive. In recent decades, as medical science trained its attention on this issue, much has changed. The birth of Louise Brown, the first "test-tube baby," on July 25, 1978, in the United Kingdom "permanently altered the prospects of fertility for many childless couples" (Braude, 1994, p.985). A new era dawned, with new options available to infertile couples. And along with new scientific advances came a host of new moral issues.

Scientific advances (more profound biological knowledge about the process of fertilization), technological changes (precision instruments that allow microsurgical procedures) and the development of new medical skills (the ability to introduce a single sperm into the cytoplasm of the oocyte) have dramatically changed our conception of human reproduction. No longer is human conception confined to the act of sexual intercourse; fertilization of a human ovum can now be done in a test tube, outside of the female body.

These developments, in the view of Snowden and Snowden (1994),

> have the potential to alter human relationships in ways that are hardly foreseeable at the present time. In terms of human reproduction western societies have embarked on a journey of almost science-fiction proportions

where parent/child, partner, kinship and even societal relationships as we know them can no longer be assumed. Presented this way, the new techniques in the treatment of infertility have epoch-making relevance at the very center of human experience (p.603).

Matters of relevance at the very center of human experience have ethical import; that is the focus of attention in the examination of some of the advances made in the new treatments of childlessness.

Is involuntary childlessness an illness which requires medical attention? Aside from a feeling of unhappiness, deep enough at times to be labeled anguish or frustration, there are no identifiable symptoms of disease. Furthermore, one can point to couples who have made a conscious decision to remain childless, yet function in a satisfactory manner within their own relationship and with society at large. A desire to have children on the part of involuntary childless couples might better be described as a want rather than a need. If that description is accepted then the question of allocation of scarce medical resources to fulfill such wants is propelled to the fore.

It can be argued, equally forcefully, that infertile couples experience distress and personal suffering as a result of their circumstances. In all societies, there is a basic assumption that the birth of children is a natural consequence of marriage or, in contemporary times where so many couples live together without formalizing the event, of a loving relationship. While some couples may be able to withstand the social and psychological pressures of childlessness, many cannot. From a medical perspective they need, and merit, intervention. In addition, all the publicity given to the new reproductive technologies has served to increase the pressure on the most vulnerable couples.

Ambivalence regarding the recognition of infertility as an illness emerges in another context, that of funding. In countries with state-funded medical plans, there is reluctance to underwrite the full costs of fertility services. Some private insurance plans include such treatments, while others do not. Braude (1994) cites the very low success rates of in vitro fertilization (IVF), and the reluctance of the state to become embroiled in the ethical, legal and social issues involved as factors influencing the lack of full funding. Another, unstated, factor could well be that the policy makers are not fully convinced that involuntary childlessness is a medical problem in the same sense as a broken leg which must be set or an inflamed appendix which must be removed. Where only partial or limited funding is available, the couple must pay the steep costs of treatment from their own funds.

IVF, as one treatment for infertility or subfertility, differs considerably in some important ways from the treatment of most other illnesses. While embarrassment may, or may not, be in the same category as ethics, it is a factor in these cases. Infertile couples have suffered sufficient anguish to motivate them to seek medical help. Exacerbating that emotion is the implicitly embarrassing admission that they no longer have reproductive liberty, which, in effect, means foregoing their autonomy to procreate naturally and in privacy. Their privacy has been invaded in a realm most people deem the most intimate of their relationship. Outside help, from physicians and scientists, is required to enable them to do what other couples pursue as a basic human function.

IVF, as a medical procedure, does not rank very high when measured in terms of success. Braude (1994) notes that although "pregnancy rates of around 25-30% per embryo transfer procedure are available, IVF still rarely results in much more than a 17% 'take home baby' rate" (p.989). Buoyed by the success of the Louise Brown case in 1978, considerable research effort has been devoted to this highly complex procedure in hopes of improving the success rate. Unfortunately very little progress has been made (Snowden and Snowden, 1994).

Additional problems beset this procedure, some medical and others ethical. "The rate of spontaneous abortion following embryo transfer is relatively high and a considerable number of pregnancies do not end in a live birth" (Snowdon and Snowdon, 1994, p.609). Achievement of a pregnancy may encourage the medical team and enhance some statistics, but unless the pregnancy results in a "take home baby," the additional harm done to the couple, in particular the woman, may far exceed any benefit unless a future pregnancy results in a live birth. Unfortunately the passage of time acts against the patient; as she gets older additional risks associated with pregnancy emerge.

One strategy employed to help overcome the low success rate is the replacement of several fertilized eggs in the mother's uterus in order to increase the chance that at least one child will be born. This strategy has resulted in a sharp increase in multiple births, as high as 300% to 400% over the past twenty years in these patients. All too often these babies are born prematurely. Many die at childbirth or very shortly thereafter, causing anguish and disappointment for the parents. Premature infants require special neonatal care, often staying in the hospital for a prolonged period of time. This places a great demand on everyone's resources, the hospital's and the parents who visit on a daily basis. A higher rate of birth defects amongst these infants than in the general population adds further complications.

Where multiple births are limited to twins or triplets the couple may get more than they anticipated but, with some guidance and assistance, they can cope. Unfortunately the number of fetuses is not always limited to two or three, or even four or five; at times the number reaches as high as eight (see Case 9.14). In such cases, all the fetuses are at risk. When such unpredicted and unwelcomed cases occur, everyone involved is forced to wrestle with the difficult ethical dilemma of selective termination.

To start the therapeutic process of IVF, a relatively large number of the woman's eggs need to be harvested, since the proportion which will be fertilized by the spermatozoa of the future mother's partner is unpredictable. To ensure an adequate supply, frequently the woman's ovaries are primed with superovulatory hormones to stimulate the development of an abundant number of follicles. This procedure can be problematic because the individual response to the stimulation regime is variable; ovarian hyperstimulation syndrome will occur in some patients. Along with a negative impact on the ovaries, other organs may be affected. Proper treatment needs to be inaugurated immediately to reverse the effects and restore the patient's health.

Due to the low success rate, more eggs are fertilized than will be replaced in the woman's ovaries. In some countries the number which can be replaced is determined by legislation; in some it is established by guidelines developed by the medical profession; and in some it is unregulated. When more embryos are available than can be replaced in the patient, an ethical problem looms large regarding the disposition of the surplus number. Cryopreservation of embryos for future use is one solution but that too can be problematic in situations where the couple divorces or one of the partners dies.

In cases where all the embryos can be frozen, the ethical problem of their final disposition has been postponed. Where not all can be frozen, a decision must be made, ethical in nature, about what to do with the surplus.

Whether surplus embryos can be used for research, as some advocate, is an ethical issue which has received considerable attention in the literature and need not be repeated here. One comment needs to be added. Mentioning research on embryos invokes the notion of personhood and the status of, in such cases, the soon-to-be fetus.

Since there are discrepancies between (1) the number of pregnancies and the number of "take home babies" and (2) the number of live births due to multiple births and the number of parents who actually take home a baby (or babies), there is flexibility (and scope) in the manner in which statistics are reported. From the perspective of the medical and scientific community, there is a need to standardize the reporting protocol so that everyone can understand precisely what is meant by the term *success rate* in this context. To benefit future patients, simplicity and clarity is required to enable them to comprehend the situation adequately prior to giving consent to proceed.

In cases where fertilized eggs cannot be replaced in the ovaries of the mother, an alternative, surrogate motherhood, is available. One woman is hired by another (or a couple) to bear a child (or children) which the first woman, for whatever reason, was unable to conceive or carry. A number of new ethical problems emerge from this "treatment regime" relating to who, really, is the mother and what the specific obligations and responsibilities are of all parties concerned.

We have not provided an exhaustive list of the ethically problematic issues emerging from the dramatic changes which have occurred in treating infertility or subfertility, rather highlighted a number of new ethical dilemmas which have arisen as a result of scientific and medical advances. The ways in which infertility can be treated now, in contrast to the very limited range of options available a short time ago, has created a new reality. Where once there was no hope, now there is some. Accompanying that hope is a host of new ethical issues which must be addressed by each practitioner involved in this realm of medicine.

Organ Transplantation

With the advent of the first successful kidney transplant in 1954, a new approach to treatment for a malfunctioning bodily organ was inaugurated. Prior to that, treatment was limited to prescribed medication or surgery. In both approaches the aim was to restore the organ to health so that it could function properly. Now, thanks to recent advances, diseased organs can be removed and replaced with other ones. As medical science has advanced, both in terms of transplantation technology and new insights into immunology, more organs are being replaced. Former hopeless conditions can now be remedied through transplantation.

The phrase "more organs are being replaced" refers to both the annual total and to the range as well. Livers, hearts, lungs and pancreases, along with kidneys, are transplanted on a regular basis. Where once, only a few years ago, each successful heart transplant was widely reported in the media as an important event, these operations are no longer considered newsworthy.

Another factor, beside scientific and medical advances, facilitated the progress made in organ transplantation. As Loewy (1989) aptly notes, "transplantation has been helped along the way by allowing brain death as the point at which death may, officially, be declared" (p.109). Since the reconceptualization of death is the topic discussed in the next section no additional comment will be made here. What needs to be highlighted is that the new line of therapy, coupled with the reconceptualization of death, have combined to create a new range of ethical issues.

Until such time as medical science solves the problems associated with transplanting animal organs into human beings, or has invented mechanical devices which can replace human organs, there are only two sources available for the procurement of replacement organs: other live human beings or the recently deceased. Each category of donor provokes ethical issues.

Organ transplantation, whether from live donors or from cadavers, has not received universal approval. A few brief comments about some of the objections to organ transplants are, therefore, in order.

The most common source of organ procurement is the newly dead. From an aesthetic and religious perspective, the thought of transplanting organs from a cadaver into a live person makes some people uncomfortable. In some religious traditions the corpse must be buried intact, with all body parts interred. Even from a non-religious perspective, removing organs from the dead can be construed as defiling the concept of wholeness and may even be regarded as mutilation. Removing organs from a cadaver may signify a lack of respect, a degradation of the individual after death into simply a source for supplying organs to the living.

In general it can be stated that the majority opinion favors harvesting organs where (1) voluntary consent has been given, either beforehand by the individual during his or her lifetime or by the immediate members of the family, and (2) where the local laws are obeyed and the medically sanctioned protocol has been followed. The benefits accruing to the recipient, from a basic utilitarian perspective (ethical judgment is rendered based on a comparison of the good and bad generated by the action in question), far outweigh any "harm" done to the cadaver.

Guidelines for the clinical determination of death have been published and circulated widely within the medical community. Protocols for determining the certainty of death have been proclaimed; pronouncements are made in those cases where there is no possibility of reversing the condition. Two physicians, experienced in the technique, separately conduct the tests on two separate occasions and their independent assessments must coincide. Furthermore, even the appearance of potential conflict of interest must be avoided. Neither physician who is conducting the tests can be attending a patient who is a potential recipient of any organ extracted from the corpse as a result of their diagnosis of brain death. Scrupulous adherence to this protocol is required since "cadaveric organ removal cannot be considered until the brain death criteria are fulfilled" (Sells, 1990, p.1009).

Where brain death criteria are not fulfilled, as in the case of a persistent vegetative state or anencephaly, organs cannot be removed. From a utilitarian perspective, the good to be gained by potential recipients from organ transplants seems to outweigh, in large measure, the bad inflicted on these unfortunate patients whose prognoses is very poor, with death inevitable. As attractive as the logic may appear to be, and as great as the potential benefits may be for the seriously ill recipients anxiously awaiting the organs, if brain death has not been pronounced, organs cannot be removed because to do so would cause the death of the patient.

At present cadaveric organs are regarded as a gift from the deceased which serves to restore the recipient to health, paving the way to a better, fuller life. That tradition is now being questioned with a view to compensating the family of the deceased donor so that they too may benefit from this altruistic act. There is a shortage of organs available for transplantation. If potential donors were aware that their next-of-kin would benefit from their decision to donate their organs, perhaps more would be inclined to sign consent forms. Implementation of that line of thinking leads to the commodification of human body parts and would, most likely, introduce entrepreneurs who would act as brokers, for a commission, between dying patients and those who need an organ to restore health.

Payment to the donor's family effectively eliminates the notion of altruism and extends commercialization into another realm of human existence. Where payment for organs becomes the accepted practice a shift in selection criteria is effected. Medical need is no longer the primary consideration; it is replaced by the ability to pay. A more frightening scenario can be sketched: a potential donor could invite bids, auctioning off organ(s) to the highest bidder. Under such circumstances, individual wealth becomes an even more important factor in determining access to health care.

Organs for transplantation, basically kidneys, can be obtained from living human beings, most often from relatives but at times from strangers. In some developing countries, India for example, the purchase of a kidney from a living donor for transplantation into a seriously ill patient who has the resources to pay is an acceptable practice. Those who agree to sell a kidney are healthy but very poor; the money received enables them, and their families, to escape the dire conditions they inhabit. A quid-pro-quo is effected: one party's health is restored and the other party's living conditions are significantly improved.

In the West, reaction to this trade in human body parts has been, to a large extent, moral outrage. The practice of selling human body parts for money has been denounced by public figures. Brecher (1990) frames the ethical issue involved: "Is payment for an organ morally acceptable? Is the buying and selling of, for example, kidneys for transplant something we should accept with (comparative) equanimity, or should we insist on donation as the only permissible form of transaction?" (p.993). These questions highlight the difference between altruism and commercialization and also direct our attention to social values as the context within which to consider these matters.

In some Western countries, the United States for example, it is commonplace for individuals to sell their blood and for patients to purchase blood when transfusions are needed. This now well-established practice is not questioned from an ethical perspective nor is anyone outraged that the practice exists. Blood removed from a healthy donor is replenished relatively quickly; hence, from a medical perspective there is little, if any, threat posed to the donor. Once a kidney is removed it will not regenerate, but it is also well known that human beings can live long, healthy lives with only one kidney. Is the difference between donating blood and donating a kidney one of kind or one only of degree? Valid arguments can be presented in support of both sides.

Payment for the purchase of bodily organs creates a market for that commodity. Commodification of bodily parts degrades us as human beings, turning us into means rather than ends. Human parts, and by logical extension, human beings, become no different from any other commodity one purchases at the supermarket or local shop. Viewed from a broader social context, this degradation could lead to a general decrease of respect for other human beings.

Where organs can be purchased for transplantation, one ethically unacceptable factor, exploitation, is likely to emerge (Campbell, Gillet and Jones, 1992). Exploitation is implicit within a market-place situation, but who is exploiting whom? Vulnerable poor healthy people, but reluctant donors, may be exploited by the lure of what to them appears to be a large sum of money. Members of the medical profession and/or their intermediaries or brokers could well be in an advantageous position to exploit the situation by catering solely to wealthy patients, who are willing to pay handsome fees for all the services needed to obtain a kidney, ahead of others whose medical conditions may be more acute.

Brecher (1990) conducts a thoughtful analysis of the propriety of selling organs for transplantation. Based on the assumption that sufficient information was supplied and that the vendor made the decision freely, autonomy was respected. Nonmaleficence is minimal since the donor can live with one kidney. Whatever little harm is done is more than adequately compensated by the benefits (beneficence); the donor/vendor receives financial benefits and the recipient/purchaser gains health benefits. In jurisdictions where the law does not prohibit such transactions, there are no legal violations. Despite the positive outcome of the analysis, Brecher maintains there is something amiss; at a more visceral level something is awry here—morally, the practice is wrong.

Perhaps the fault lies in choosing medical ethical principles as the framework within which to conduct the analysis. A more pertinent context may be a particular society's vision of the good life and how its poor people are treated. A society which condones the practice of selling organs has either insufficient regard for the poor or insufficient resources to distribute to ensure that they need not resort to such practices to escape poverty.

Given that there is an insufficient supply of donor organs, is a society morally justified in prohibiting the sale of bodily organs which, in effect, means that patients who desperately need them are condemned to die? How each individual responds to this ethical dilemma will, in part, reflect personal values and a specific model of medical practice. A physician committed totally to prolonging the life of a patient may be more inclined to approve the practice of paying for organs, since more will be available, thereby keeping more patients alive. Another physician, whose concern encompasses an overview of the values held by society, in particular how it treats its poor, may be more inclined to condemn such a practice.

Voluntarily donating an organ to a relative is an altruistic act of great magnitude. Is this truly the case in all situations? Watching the suffering of a renal patient near the end stage can be a heart-wrenching experience. Witnessing such agony may motivate a close relative to volunteer a kidney. It could be posited that the stress placed on the donor by his or her love for the ailing relative can be regarded as compulsion. Where compulsion to donate is present it seems to eliminate or at least diminish the notion of altruism. However, it is important to remember that the potential donor retains autonomy and can decide to proceed or refuse to donate the organ. If the decision is to proceed, then it could be argued, equally forcefully, that a greater degree of altruism is present.

Another ethical dilemma emerging as a result of the shortage of available kidneys merits brief consideration. At times, criminals condemned to death volunteer their organs for transplantation after they are executed. Other criminals, serving long sentences, may volunteer a kidney as a means of partially atoning for the crime committed. In both situations, the source of the donation comes under close scrutiny. Is it proper to accept human organs from an "evil" source? Some argue that no matter how important it is to increase the supply, organs from criminals are tainted and therefore should not be used. Others argue, perhaps with greater force, that they should be accepted, since the organs are not tainted and using them will save the lives of patients who otherwise will die.

New science, new technology, new clinical practice and a new conceptualization of therapy (replacing diseased organs with healthy ones from a donor) has helped countless patients but, at the same time, has created new ethical dilemmas in both developing and advanced societies.

Death and Dying

Death is final. There is a sharp demarcation between life and death; once the line has been crossed, there is no return. As Shakespeare wrote in Hamlet, death is "the undiscovered country from whose bourn no traveler returns." We have respect for the living and we have respect for the dead because they were once live human beings. However, there is a difference in the treatment accorded the living and the treatment accorded the dead, due to their position on one side or the other of the dividing line. From both a legal and an ethical stance, there are things we can do to living human beings that we cannot do to corpses, and, conversely, there are things we can do to corpses that we cannot do to living human beings.

In the past there was one standard used for determining death. "For thousands of years, definitions of death focused on cessation of breathing and heartbeat. When breathing stopped, cardiac anoxia (lack of oxygen to an area) and ischemia (lack of blood flow to an area) resulted, causing the heart to stop" (Pence, 1990, p.17). Under this conception lay people could tell when death occurred: when the tangible evidence of life, breathing and heartbeat, were no longer present for some time, everyone knew the person had died.

The practice of medicine experienced major changes in the 1950s and 1960s leading to innovative procedures and, perhaps more important, new thinking about what achievements were possible. Human organs could be transplanted, starting with the first successful kidney transplant in 1954, and then, with Dr. Barnard's pioneering work in 1967, with heart transplants. Improved technology, new approaches to treatment, and scientific advances made a significant difference: "ventilators and ICUs changed things, allowing artificial respiration of brain-damaged patients" (Pence, 1990, p.17). Technology, combined with a more profound understanding of human biology, enabled physicians to keep a patient's body functioning long after the brain had suffered severe damage as a result of trauma or oxygen deprivation. Somatic function could be maintained even after the irreversible loss of consciousness. Important new insights emerged, including:

> the awareness that intervention could make it possible to prevent the brain from succumbing to cardiac and respiratory arrest on the one hand, and make it possible, on the other hand, artificially to maintain the heartbeat and circulation of the blood in a body whose brain had ceased to function as an integrated whole. In short: the natural link between the function of the brain and the heart and lungs had been severed (Lamb, 1994, p.1035).

At the same time, the need to harvest more human organs for transplantation became apparent. Since the validity of donor organs diminishes quickly once circulation ceases, comatose patients whose somatic functions are continued by artificial means (respirators) become highly desirable sources of organs for transplantation. This knowledge, implicitly or sometimes overtly, exerted pressure to rethink the status of patients with irreversible, severe brain damage.

Rethinking the status of patients with irreversible severe brain damage in essence meant rethinking the concept of death itself. As Lamb (1994) points out, "[the] way forward lay in considering the importance of the brain. Notwithstanding the emotional significance of the heart the significance of the brain as both the unit of consciousness and cognition, and as the organizing faculty of the body 'as a whole', has long been recognized" (p.1035). Cessation of brain function, rather than cessation of cardiorespiratory function, could serve as the criterion for death. In 1968 the ad hoc committee of Harvard Medical School published its report recommending whole brain death as the standard. Death, as a concept, had been reconceptualized.

The reconceptualization of death evokes questions about two issues mentioned previously, personhood, and the distinction between sanctity of life and quality of life. It could be posited that a cardiorespiratory definition of death focuses more on the somatic notion of personhood and on the sanctity of life. So long as the patient is breathing, whether in an irreversible coma or not, that person is alive and everything ought to be done to prolong that life. In contrast, a brain-death definition of death directs attention to the psychological aspects (without disregarding the soma) of personhood and evokes the notion of quality of life. This definition of death acknowledges the importance of consciousness and personality as ontological components of personhood. In effect, a person is more than a body. Where there are no signs of brain activity, consciousness is absent; when this state is irreversible, the notion of personhood is difficult to sustain.

Death as a concept appears to defy precise definition, nor, it seems, has one standard measurement been accepted by the medical community. Pence (1990) notes that there are four basic standards: whole-body, whole-brain, irreversible unconsciousness and higher brain. Each standard has its own supporters and detractors and each has a set of ethical issues associated with it. One issue common to all is the need for certainty before pronouncing death.

Technological changes coupled with advancements in medical care, particularly in ICUs, have compelled not only the medical community but all persons to achieve a better understanding of death. Along with greater understanding is a need, even in face of the difficulty, to define death. In this regard it is important to note Lamb's (1990) caution: "The definition of death is primarily a philosophical and moral matter. This is because technical data alone cannot answer purely conceptual questions" (p.1028). An important addition to this comment, many would insist, is the need for theological consideration. Technical data is needed to help everyone understand the biological functions as well as the interrelationship between biology and psychology, but as the study evolves, the clearer the claim becomes that this is a philosophical and moral matter.

Under the cardiorespiratory concept of death, or whole-body death, matters were somewhat more straightforward and the standards were somewhat clearer. With the advent of the three other standards, whole-brain, irreversible unconsciousness, and higher brain, death become more complicated and what was once a seemingly simple question to answer now becomes problematic. Under the cardiorespiratory concept of death, a reply to the question "When did death occur?" can most often be given—just after the person drew his or her last breath. When the other standards are invoked the answer to that question becomes problematic.

Since what can be done ethically and legally to a living person differs from what can be done to a corpse, a clear answer to when death occurs is needed. Modern technology can maintain cardiorespiratory function indefinitely, even when there is no brain activity. Under the whole-body conception of death these persons would be considered alive, yet under the whole-brain conception these same persons could be pronounced dead. Using technology to maintain cardiorespiratory function creates problems: "the beating heart cadaver" (Lamb, 1994, p.1034) blurs the boundary between life and death. This phenomenon has distressed physicians as well as relatives of the supposed deceased.

This problem, which affects everyone involved, is phrased succinctly by Campbell, et al. (1992): "It seems that we can say that a person's life has ended when that person enters irreversible coma, even though the illusion that he is alive might persist and indeed be sustained for a while" (p.111). When did death occur? Was it at the moment of the onset of irreversible coma, even though the heart continued to beat? Or was it when the qualified physicians completed their tests and made their pronouncement? Or was it when the patient was finally removed from the ventilator?

Complicating matters is the need for still-viable organs for transplantation. Hence, careful philosophical consideration needs to be devoted to clarifying the standards of whole-brain, irreversible unconsciousness, and higher brain death. A transplant is more likely to succeed if organs are removed immediately after death has been pronounced. Maintaining a supply of blood and oxygen to the organs of the potential donor prevents deterioration from setting in; therefore, maintaining the cardiorespiratory function for as long as possible, or as near as possible to the time death is pronounced, is most desirable. As important as these factors are, the first consideration from an ethical perspective must be given to the dying patient.

There are important differences with regard to the medical status and notions of personhood between the standards applied to the whole-brain, irreversible unconsciousness, and higher brain conceptions of death. In some jurisdictions, legal standards apply, but when there are no laws regulating practice, the need for serious ethical consideration becomes much more important.

A disturbing aspect of human dying in contemporary times is noted by Escobar (1990). Modern medical practice and new technology is serving to prolong the process of dying. Physicians are no longer allowing a natural process, as sad or as unwanted as it may seem, to happen. What is being prolonged is the patient's purely biological life, while the agony of the members of the family is also prolonged. Since many more patients are dying in hospitals, whereas before they died at home, more resources are being used. Death is final; with it comes grieving and then closure. In raising this matter, Escobar invites us to address another ethical facet of how scientific and technological advances have affected the treatment of death and dying.

A quarter of a century after the issuance of the Harvard Medical School report, and despite the wide acceptance given to the notion of brain-death, there are still dissenters. M. Evans (1994), a philosopher who wrote a paper entitled "Against Brainstem Death," starts his objection from the position that "the human body is worthy of moral concern and respect even in death; it matters morally how we treat the dead" (p.1041). He then proceeds to argue that in any definition of death what we, as ordinary lay people and medical personnel see, may have more force than theoretical or abstract definitions. In his view, the presence of heartbeat is a critical factor and cannot be dismissed as is done by those who support a brain-death conception of death. For Evans, the prolonged cessation of heartbeat is the criterion for death.

Taking advantage of his position as editor, R. Gillon (1994) sets out to refute Evans' stand. He proceeds by attempting to show the weaknesses in some of the arguments and, to a much larger extent, by offering a medical explanation about the function of the brain and its role in controlling and regulating the organs and processes within the body. From a medical perspective it would be very difficult to disagree with Gillon, but that is not quite the case regarding what he cites as a serious weakness in one of the arguments used by Evans. Gillon rejects the view put forward by Evans who avers that the everyday concept of being alive is the presence of a heartbeat and a warm body; conversely the absence of a heartbeat and a cold, clammy appearance are signs of death. Gillon objects to Evans' reliance on the strategy of utilizing common usage and commonly accepted views. That is always a dicey ploy since common usage and commonly accepted views are amenable to an array of interpretations.

As strong as Gillon's stance may appear on the medical explanation, there is room to question the validity of his riposte regarding commonly accepted views. A middle position between the two will be sketched, and then some empirical evidence will be offered to support Evans. Within the medical world, with its own culture and its advanced scientific comprehension of human biology, the notion of brain-death as the valid conception of death is readily understood and hence accepted. This concept, or set of concepts, has not been transmitted to the general populace; they have not been educated along these new lines, neither in school where death is rarely, if ever, considered, nor by the medical community through the mass media. It could be posited that what most people know about death has been transmitted to them from within their extended families, and, as has been noted earlier, for centuries the generally accepted conception of death was the cessation of the cardiorespiratory function.

A case reported in *The Ottawa Citizen* (Waiting for a miracle, February 15, 1997, B1, B4) lends support to the stand taken by Evans regarding the primacy of heartbeat as an indicator of life. Competent, experienced physicians had prepared the family of a ten-year-old girl to accept the futility of their daughter's situation. A malignant tumor was growing in her brain. As she lay in the ICU, hooked to life support systems, the parents were told by the physician that, sadly, she was dead. All that needed to be done was to turn off the respirator. The mother, a deeply religious woman, responded in no uncertain terms: unhooking their daughter would be murder. The family's pastor nodded his head in agreement. Despite all the efforts by various medical personnel to convince the parents, they would not accept their daughter's death so long as her heart kept beating.

There is more to this sad tale. The daughter was taken home eventually, and the insurance company, although notified by the hospital that, in their view, the girl was dead, agreed to pay the costs for an array of health care professionals who attended her. On two occasions the mother succeeded in having her daughter admitted to another hospital for surgery to remove tissue obstructing ventilation. Fourteen months after she was first declared brain-dead, the girl's heart gave out, and then it was over.

Although this episode is offered as some support for the position taken by Evans, and as a minor argument against Gillon, its major function is to call our attention to that vital question: When did death occur? Which conception of death is acceptable? On what basis do we accept one and reject the others? While there is a medical basis required for the replies, the queries posed are philosophical in nature and the replies obviously carry great ethical import.

The Need for Education in Ethics

Incoming medical practitioners, those of the past as well as the most recent graduates, have sworn an oath as part of the graduation ritual. As noted earlier, these oaths are ethical in nature and serve, in a clear way, to indicate the moral component of all aspects of medical practice. Loewy (1989) points out that "ethics is an integral part of the fabric of medical decision making and has undoubtedly always been an important consideration in medical practice" (p.2). Recent technological and scientific advances have brought many benefits to countless patients but have also served to propel the ethical component of medicine to greater prominence. An additional consequence of these advances is to underscore the need on the part of all health care practitioners for more knowledge about ethics to complement their more scientifically and technologically sophisticated practice.

Medicine, along with many other professions, can accurately be described as a decision-making activity. As the examination of a patient proceeds, decisions are being made constantly regarding which questions to ask, which procedures to employ, which tests to order, what possible diagnosis to make and which medication to prescribe. A multitude of factors are taken into consideration: the patient and his or her needs, the family, potential costs involved and resources available, to mention but a few. Some of the decisions can be made almost entirely on the basis of scientific fact and medical evidence, but many other issues fall outside that realm. This latter category, often ethical in nature, needs to be addressed from a philosophical perspective, but it must also take into account the scientific and medical factors. Neither the scientific approach by itself nor the philosophic approach by itself is adequate to address the issues in these cases. A multidisciplinary approach is required.

Any time there is interaction between persons, as in the case of the health care professional and patient, there are questions, ethical in nature, about how these persons ought to act. Each person has obligations to the other, and how those obligations are discharged is open to ethical scrutiny. It is assumed that each health care professional not only desires to act ethically but will do so at all times. Given the array of complex and confounding ethical dilemmas that each professional practitioner will likely confront, good intentions alone are insufficient. Knowledge and analytical skills are required as the basis and tool needed for making proper decisions.

One thing is certain in health care: ethical dilemmas will emerge. Attempting to deal with each situation as it arises, on a case-by-case basis, will prove to be difficult and frustrating since there is no foundation upon which to base a decision. To confound matters, it is unlikely that there will be "text book cases" that are amenable to standard solutions. Deciding moral questions, in all realms of health care—practice, technology, research—requires a moral framework; that framework is usually called an ethical theory.

Ethical dilemmas cannot be avoided. It would be advantageous to have developed a reasoned moral stance before proceeding with any decision or action. Arriving at that position requires knowledge of some ethical theories and the development of critical and analytical skills based on a rational thought process. In all realms of human activity, more knowledge is better than less. So it is with practice in health care, only in this realm, knowledge is needed in both the technical and ethical components. The technical component (both the theoretical and practical) is well covered in the various curricula, but the same cannot be said for the ethical component (Baylis and Downie, 1990), which needs more attention. The succeeding chapters of this book are devoted to strengthening that component—both the theoretical and applied—of the education of health care professionals.

3

Introduction to Ethics

As stated previously, there are two indissoluble component parts, the technical and the ethical, to all practice in health care. When addressing any situation it is important to ponder both components thoroughly, be it within the framework of professional practitioner-patient relationship, or the hospital/treatment institution-patient relationship, or the professional practitioner-professional practitioner relationship. An overemphasis on the technical component, while disregarding the ethical implications or consequences, may achieve some therapeutic goals, but the social costs involved may negate whatever benefits are gained. Conversely, there may be occasions when a discussion of the fine points of ethics needs to be set aside in favor of immediate medical intervention. There appears to be very little, if any, likelihood of such a situation actually occurring. However, there are a sufficient number of instances of the former sort reported to merit reminding practitioners to consider the ethical component routinely as a matter of standard procedure.

Axiological Framework

Health care practitioners, as individual professionals striving to improve their practice, spend some time reviewing their treatment of patients and their interaction with colleagues, be it members of their own specialty or members of other specialties or administrators. Along with an assessment of the technical component—the diagnosis made, the tests ordered, and the treatment prescribed—there is also an examination of the non-technical component. Were the rules followed? Was the patient accorded proper respect and consideration as a person? Were the institution's policies adhered to? Were colleagues treated properly? Did I behave in a way which is consonant with my own nature and set of values?

Reflection and introspection are integral components of professional practice and important procedures to ensure continued improvement. Looking back to ponder judgments rendered and actions taken necessarily involves a review of the technical component as well as the ethical component. In one sense the technical component is more readily measured: Did the patient recover? Was the recovery uneventful? Did it occur within the usual time frame for that illness or trauma? It is the examination of the non-technical component, focusing on human relationships and interactions, that provides the axiological (value-laden) framework. In this realm, ethics, values and norms are brought to the fore.

Basic Concepts and Definitions

It may seem redundant to provide definitions for such common terms as ethics, morals, values and norms, since these words are often used in everyday speech. Ironically, it is because of the widespread use—and misuse at times—of these terms that they have taken on many meanings thus indicating a need for the provision of definitions to standardize our understanding. Definitions are provided, along with pertinent elaboration, to clarify current usage and to provide additional insights into the axiological framework. Understandings derived from the definitions will facilitate the reading of the text.

Values are those deeply held views that serve to motivate and guide our behavior. A value is an enduring belief that a particular way of behaving and living is personally and socially preferable to other ways of behaving and living. Values are enduring qualities that set out the path of life we follow. Values can be positive or negative, depending on the person's perspective. While the word *value*, like ethics and morals, covers the gamut of behavior from good to bad, when used as a descriptor it generally has a positive connotation.

Norms refer to standards or generally held sets of criteria (*norms* is a contraction of the term *normative*). We can use these criteria as a maxim or measuring rod against which to assess behavior. Norms, used in conjunction with judgments (about actions, about how people should behave, about values, and about which goals are worth pursuing), provide this framework.

Ethics is an acknowledged branch of philosophy. As the word is commonly used, *ethics* is concerned with issues of right and wrong in human conduct; it is concerned with what is good and what is bad, what is authentic and what is inauthentic. Ethics is also concerned with the notions of duty, obligation and moral responsibility. As such, ethics are manifested in behavior and assessed through the application of ethical inquiry, which utilizes critical moral reasoning.

An understanding of what is, and what ought to be, is basic to assessing behavior. In order to assess behavior, either what is or what has occurred, as a basis for rendering moral judgments we need to know what is right, what is good and what is authentic. Although the three terms, right, good and authentic, refer to ethical standards or ideals, there are differences between them. Generally, we employ the terms right and wrong in situations where rules and laws are applicable; we use the terms good and bad when attention is focused on the consequences of the act; and, we apply the terms authentic and inau-

Figure 3.1: Axiological Framework: The Interrelationship between Values, Norms, and Ethics

VALUES	NORMS	ETHICS
Individual beliefs which motivate and guide behavior.	Group or societal standards or generally held criteria for acceptable conduct.	Objective basis upon which judgments are rendered regarding right or wrong, good or bad, authentic or inauthentic behavior.

thentic to situations where an individual critically examines his or her own behavior. Additional information regarding these differences is provided later in the chapter, in the section entitled Three Ethical Bases.

From a disciplinary perspective, ethics, as the study of morals, refers to that branch of philosophy which critically examines, clarifies and reframes the basic concepts and presuppositions of ethical theories and of morality generally. In contemporary times this branch of philosophy has been roughly organized into two categories, metaethics and applied ethics. Metaethics is more theoretical in nature, as scholars involved in this work train their sights on the logic, coherence and presuppositions found in each ethical theory. In contrast, as the title suggests, applied ethics is much more concerned with examining behavior to determine if a specific act is right or wrong, good or bad, authentic or inauthentic.

Both metaethics and applied ethics interrelate at the level of theory and practice. Ethical theory must be grounded in actual human existence, for if that were not so, it would be difficult to imagine its applicability. And, since moral judgment is rendered based on some standard or ethical maxim, an ethical theory is necessarily invoked.

Ethics, values and *norms* combine to form the axiological framework (Figure 3.1). Additional discussion of this topic is found in Chapter 8 where the five medical principles and various models of medical practice are presented.

Morals is the term more often used when referring to actions, behavior and the principles that guide them. Technically speaking, from a disciplinary perspective, morality is a central concept of ethics but it is not the totality of that study. Morality often refers to certain principles which seem to make absolute and universal claims (e.g., thou shalt not steal). In contemporary times, *moral* is usually the term applied to an individual's actions although there are times when ethics is the descriptor used. Through moral categories we can judge if a particular act was right or wrong, good or bad, virtuous or evil, authentic or inauthentic.

Two features of the terms *ethics* and *morals*, as they are currently used, merit highlighting. First, most often *ethical* and *moral* are interchangeable terms. An ethical issue is a moral issue; a moral issue is an ethical issue. Second, both terms, *ethical* and *moral*, can be used in two distinctly different ways. In one way, both terms cover the full gamut of appraisals, ranging from absolute good, right, or virtue, to absolute bad, wrong or evil, with various shades of gray between. When these terms are used in this manner it is the aim of the speaker or writer to direct our attention to a particular feature, the ethical or moral component, of the behavior in question. We are invited to focus on the rightness or wrongness of the action. Within this context, ethics and morals are used interchangeably to refer to good and proper behavior and to bad and improper behavior. We say that someone who constantly violates the rules has the ethics or morals of an alley cat. Yet, if someone behaves in an exemplary fashion, we call that behavior ethical or moral. The terms *ethical* and *moral* are used in still another way. When used to describe the behavior or motivation of a person, it will be a positive comment meaning right or good, in keeping with common usage.

Medical ethics, **bioethics** and **biomedical ethics** are three terms applied to the realm of health care (Barry, 1982; Williams, 1986). Each descriptor is meant to designate a specific area of human activity as the focus of concern and object of moral scrutiny. As such, the term *medical ethics* can be interpreted to mean that the focus is narrowly confined to the practice of medicine; *bioethics* would enlarge the scope somewhat to include a number of sciences associated with the practice of medicine; and *biomedical ethics* designates the widest range, encompassing the complex of moral issues which arise in medical practice (here interpreted broadly to include all the members of the multidisciplinary team, such as nursing, physiotherapy and speech therapy, as examples) and emerge in the research fields associated with medicine and health care. These three terms are often used interchangeably in the literature, covering the entire gamut of practice, therapy, administration and research.

Biomedical ethics is an applied branch of ethics which links ethics with biomedicine. As such it is guided by the tenets and rules found in various ethical theories and utilizes critical moral reasoning when attempts are made to assess behavior and render moral judgment in the realm of health care.

The practice of biomedical ethics is akin to the practice of applied ethics in other realms of human conduct, such as sport and business. However, certain circumstances prevail in health care which invite special consideration. Much of the attention in biomedical ethics is focused on the patient, a sick person who is in need of treatment. At these times the patient is more vulnerable; hence, the amount of trust placed in the health care practitioner is greater than it is in other client-professional relationships. A higher degree of trust, in the view of many, places a greater onus on the practitioner to demonstrate more

Figure 3.2: Focus of Ethical Theory

DEONTOLOGY	TELEOLOGY	EXISTENTIALISM
Behavior based upon what is **Right**.	Behavior based upon what is **Good**.	Behavior based upon what is **Authentic**.

sensitivity to all the needs of the patient during treatment. What under other circumstances would be deemed minor, relatively inconsequential indiscretions, loom much larger when a person's health or life is at stake. These considerations may place biomedical ethics in a somewhat different category from other branches of applied ethics.

Three Ethical Bases

Throughout history, serious thinkers have explored and proposed a wide range of sources as bases for ethics. These bases are often called *ethical theories*. Some proposed sources include the good life, self-interest, the love of God, respect for persons, duty, the greatest good for the greatest number, sympathy, social justice, using a scientific approach to assess behavior and radical freedom (existentialism). Some approaches have persisted over time as generally accepted bases for ethics. Three are of particular interest (Figure 3.2). A brief introductory comment on each is presented here to serve as the basis for a more extensive discussion in the next chapter.

Approach 1. A rule-based approach, focusing on obligation and duty, similar to the orientation found in the Bible. Since attention is directed to the act itself, this approach is non-consequentialist. Technically, the term used is *deontology*.

Approach 2. An approach that focuses on the consequences of the action, one that conceives of ethics as concerned with measuring the amount of goodness, or badness, arising from behavior. Attention is directed toward assessing the consequences of a particular action rather than examining the act itself. Technically, the term used is *teleology*.

Approach 3. In contemporary times, under the influence of post-World War II European thought (which includes philosophy and Third Force psychology), attention was directed squarely at the individual. Concepts such as authenticity, which refers to how true the person is to him or herself, integrity and genuineness are factors that must be considered in judging each individual act at that particular time within the context of the unique, prevailing circumstances. Technically, the term used is *existentialism*.

Each of the three bases and/or approaches listed above identifies a source from which we derive ethical maxims. Problems can, and usually will, arise during moral discourse if there is no explicit agreement reached regarding which ethical maxim will serve as the yardstick or standard against which to measure behavior. Using different ethical bases can lead to divergent judgments. An example will serve to illustrate this.

> Jane Doe, a thirty-something business executive, telephoned from out of town to book an appointment with her family physician (Dr. A) for the next day, immediately following her arrival home. She was bothered by acute symptoms of vaginal discharge and dysuria. An examination and tests confirmed a sexually transmitted disease (STD). She confessed that it was an impetuous act while away at this business conference; it was a one-time occurrence and totally out of character with her usual behavior. As luck would have it, her husband had left town on a business trip of his own the day before she returned. Dr. A looked after both husband and wife.

> Jane was aware that the law in her political jurisdiction required physicians to report all cases of sexually transmitted diseases to the local health council. Jane Doe pleaded with Dr. A not to report her case or inform her husband since it would pose a serious threat to their marriage. With proper treatment, she expected her condition to clear up completely before her husband returned. Married life would continue on blissfully in the same way as it had prior to her trip.

If a ruled-based orientation is used as the source of the ethical maxim and Dr. A does not report the case, the physician's behavior would be wrong. If one takes a consequentialist's approach, assuming that the medication prescribed clears up the condition completely prior to the husband's return, and the case is not reported, greater good or happiness would result—the marriage would be preserved—from not reporting the case. From an existential perspective, Jane Doe would need to examine her conscience to determine if asking someone to break a law for her benefit is an authentic act. As well, Dr. A would need to search her conscience to decide if, by not reporting the case, she is being true to herself.

Ethical Bases (Theories) and Values Clarification

Three different sources of ethical bases have been briefly sketched, and ethical maxims can be derived from each of them. As illustrated in the case of Jane Doe, the behavior under scrutiny can be assessed from all three ethical bases and, on occasion, somewhat surprisingly, contrary ethical judgments can be rendered. This creates a new problem which needs to be addressed: Which of the three moral judgments do we accept and which do we reject?

Confronting this problem requires, among other things, the clarification of your own values. Do you regard obeying the rules as more important than evaluating the goodness (and badness) resulting from an action? Or do you subscribe to the view that the end justifies the means, particularly in situations where the end creates more goodness than badness? If this is your belief, are you prepared to break rules in cases where, on balance, you predict more goodness than badness will result from your actions? How important is it for you to be authentic, to behave in a way that is consistent with what you truly believe?

When faced with a choice, which is most important for you: Obeying the rules under all circumstances? Or is it making certain that the results of your action produces more goodness than badness, no matter the behavior used to attain that goal? Or is it maintaining authenticity, that is, being true to yourself at all times without regard for adherence to the rules and possible outcomes regarding goodness and badness? As you rank these options in order of your personal preference, you are engaging in a values clarification exercise through which you will (1) learn more about yourself and (2) obtain some insights into which ethical base (theory), deontology (rules, non-consequential), teleology (outcome, consequential) or existentialism (authenticity) is more likely to influence your thinking and moral reasoning.

Moral Discourse and Moral Reasoning

Differences of opinion over moral issues have probably existed since our forbears began interacting with each other. A review of contemporary writing, in all fields, reveals disagreement and controversy between professional practitioners, philosophers, theologians and members of the public. We cannot expect to find unanimity in ethics and in moral judgments except on rare occasions. When we do find agreement, it occurs mostly when the exhibited behavior is at either of the extreme ends of the moral spectrum. Behavior that contains minimal ethical content is rarely subject to scrutiny or cause for dispute. Since we readily reach agreement in such cases without serious discussion, very little is learned. Similarly, blatant, obviously immoral acts provoke little, if any, moral disagreement. In such cases, discussion tends to focus on the motivation that prompted the act or on the sanctions to be applied.

Between these two extremes are countless acts that invite moral judgment. Ethical dilemmas emerge daily in every facet of professional practice; incidents and events that demand moral scrutiny. When we begin discussing these incidents and assessing behavior we are engaged in doing ethics. Doing ethics involves judging human beings in terms of ends or goals attained as well as the means used to achieve them. Included in this approach is an examination of the relationship between the means and the ends. Doing ethics involves using data, and it also requires techniques of describing, analyzing, assessing, judging and making decisions.

Examining data critically in order to render judgment is part of a process called moral reasoning. Moral reasoning is a systematic approach that enables us to probe deeply in order to see things with greater clarity. It frees us from dogmatic and prejudiced thinking. Freedom from dogmatic and prejudiced thinking creates intellectual independence. Issues and statements are analyzed critically using rational thought in place of emotional appeal. An integral part of moral reasoning is the requirement to provide reasons to support the position taken or the moral judgment rendered.

The provision of reasons places the discussion above the level of mere opinion. If the discussion remains at the level of mere opinion little, if any, advancement or progress is made. When reasons are offered in support of the view expressed, the impasse can be broken. Once reasons are offered, they can be evaluated and weighed in terms of their pertinence, cogency and force. By comparing the total strength of the reasons provided in support of one view to the total force of a contrary view, a determination can be made about which is the more logical and/or stronger argument.

Through a critical examination of the reasons given, faulty logic, inconsistent thinking and inapplicable rationales can be detected. Disciplined, impartial, logical thinking is required in order to criticize the reasons given and to ferret out discrepancies. This analytical process, difficult and arduous at times, leads to greater moral insights, thus placing the dialogue well beyond the realm of mere opinion. Based on rational thought and sound reasoning, moral judgments rendered through this process are apt to better withstand criticism.

Moral reasoning is not conducted as an exercise in abstract thought. As applied ethics, moral reasoning aims to identify and delineate right conduct and correct behavior. As we explore and analyze the cases in Chapter 8, we become aware of the moral options available to us as well as the wide range of ethical dilemmas which are encountered as real-life issues. Another lesson emerges, particularly in cases where divergent ethical judgments are rendered: caution must be used before declaring an action absolutely right or absolutely wrong, absolutely good or absolutely bad. There are shades of gray inherent in the judgment of human conduct.

Moral reasoning is a skill which needs to be acquired. Like all other skills, practice, often guided by a more knowledgeable person, is required in order to improve one's ability. Ample opportunity to practice moral reasoning skills is provided in Chapter 9, where a wide array of case studies are found.

Agent Accountability

A person is accountable for his or her actions. Technically, we identify that person as an agent. To understand what it means to be accountable requires an understanding of what it means to be an agent. An agent has free will and the power to act. Having free will and the power to act allows the agent to choose, from among options, which action to perform. By choosing to act in a certain way, an agent accepts responsibility for that action and its consequences. An agent is accountable for actions done intentionally; here we link account- ability to intention, which is an integral part of the action. Involuntary actions and accidental actions are generally placed in another moral category. Both motivation and intention are not always obvious. Difficulties may be encoun- tered in determining the status of motivation and intention in the act.

Model I—Basic Approach

To guide the flow of moral discourse, two models are presented, one here and the second in Chapter 5. This first model (Figure 3.3), more basic in nature, is designed primarily to facilitate and guide deliberation when the cases in Chapter 9 are examined. It offers a logical progression which, if followed, will ensure comprehensive treatment of the issues involved. This model can be used to examine all behavior from an ethical perspective.

Step One—Obtain and Clarify All the Pertinent Facts

To ensure that everyone involved in the discussion is operating from the same base, it is important that all the facts be presented. Everyone needs to know exactly what happened. This advice is proffered with full awareness of the warning issued by Francoeur (1983) and Veatch (1977) about the impossi- bility of presenting all the information needed for a complete analysis of each case. Some facts may be missing, but sufficient information about each case found in Chapter 9 is presented to permit a comprehensive discussion.

The incident or event must be considered not only in proper chronological order, but also in terms of who was present, their roles, responsibilities and the understandings (both tacit and explicit) that prevailed then. This procedure is similar to the evidence being presented at a trial in court. In order for the judge and jury to arrive at a just verdict, all the facts of the case need to be presented, along with as much background and context as possible. The same line of thinking applies to moral reasoning.

Step Two—Identify and Enunciate the Ethical Maxim(s) to Be Used

An ethical maxim is a general moral principle, rule, law or moral doctrine that one adopts or formulates to serve as a yardstick against which behavior

Figure 3.3: Model I—A Five-Step Approach for Rendering Ethical Judgment

1. Obtain and clarify all the pertinent facts of the case or incident.

2. Identify and enunciate the ethical maxim(s). This is the standard against which the behavior/action/incident/event is measured.

3. Time.

4. Identify and discuss any extenuating circumstances.

5. Render judgment.

can be measured. It can be understood as a moral rule of thumb and, as such, it can also serve to guide behavior.

Omission of this step will likely add confusion, as the use of different implicit maxims will create a situation where people talk past each other. Once an ethical maxim has been enunciated, it serves to direct the discussion along one agreed-upon path of moral reasoning; everyone involved understands the yardstick being used as the measuring rod.

As explained earlier, the three ethical theories, deontology, teleology and existentialism, are sources from which ethical maxims can be derived. From a deontological perspective the following questions can be asked: Are there any specific rules which apply? Are there any "unwritten" but generally accepted procedures which are pertinent? Do any of the policies of the institution cover the issue at hand? Are there broader social standards which can be invoked? Do any of the laws of that particular jurisdiction apply? If there is a rule governing that behavior then that rule serves as an ethical maxim. In such cases the rule may apply in two realms, the legal and the moral. If no rule is applicable, the next step may be to consult the institution's policies and procedures. Generally speaking, it is easier to arrive at a consensus where explicit rules or clear statements are available. A consensus is more difficult to obtain in the realm of "unwritten" rules and social standards since these areas are amenable to a wider array of interpretation.

A teleological (consequentialist) approach focuses on the end results produced. Did that particular action generate more good than bad? Ethical maxims, formulated within this context, will be phrased in a way that allows for the comparison of benefits (goods) and drawbacks (bad) resulting from the action. This is one of the basic issues in euthanasia. Attempting such calculations is a difficult challenge, since goodness and badness are not readily amenable to quantification. Estimates can be made of the impact the action is likely to have on everyone involved in that particular event. This step assists us in calculating the sum total of good and the sum total of bad resulting from the incident.

Consideration given to the greatest good for the greatest number serves as a general guide in public policy, but that notion is more difficult to apply to individuals. Despite this caveat, we can often determine if an event had a minimal or a major impact. In calculating the sum of goodness and the sum of badness, consideration needs to be given to both quantity and quality; some events have a more profound impact than others.

From an existential perspective, the focus is trained on the person, with two characteristics, authenticity and genuineness, coming to the fore. Authenticity is a characteristic based on the concept of congruence: congruence within the person (affective and cognitive domains) and congruence between the person, the person's actions and the world. A person is authentic to the degree to which the person's being in the world is unqualifiedly in accord with the basis of that person's own nature and own conception of the world. An authentic person thinks, feels and acts in a consistent, congruent manner. Authenticity is a personal matter. Only the person can know the authenticity of his or her being. To be genuine, honest, congruent or real means to be authentic to oneself. The person is the only one who can know what is going on inside the self. Genuineness reflects the authenticity of each person.

The search for an ethical maxim cannot be conducted in isolation, separate and apart from the incident under scrutiny. Step Two cannot be the exclusive focus of attention; some consideration needs to be given to Step One at the same time. Kantor (1989) states that "individual cases often have many layers of conflict, if only because there are usually many persons involved in the case.... They may have different perspectives, and there may be a number of types of obligations and rights involved in their interactions" (p.33). This comment helps to explain why it may be difficult, at times, to select one ethical maxim that is acceptable to everyone.

More than one ethical maxim can be found to serve as the moral yardstick against which behavior can be measured. Recall the case involving Jane Doe. She asked her physician to disregard the law which calls for the reporting of all sexually transmitted diseases to the local health council and pleaded with her not to inform her husband in order to avoid a crisis in the marriage. In such situations, more than one ethical maxim can be identified. It is possible to apply more than one ethical maxim to the act/incident/event in question. Invoking more than one ethical maxim promotes a wider-ranging moral discourse. A more comprehensive examination of the behavior/act/incident/event is preferable to a narrower review, since the former produces greater insights and, therefore more, rather than less, ethical knowledge.

Step Three—Time

Chronologically we can look to (1) the time before the incident, (2) the time of the incident and (3) the consequences that resulted because of the incident. In the quest for a comprehensive description of what occurred, it is usually advantageous to know what prompted the action under examination. That knowledge often helps us to understand the act itself. Knowing precisely, and in detail, what happened when the incident occurred adds to the foundation upon which moral reasoning is conducted. Assessing the consequences helps us to determine the gravity or severity of the situation. As the moral reasoning exercise evolves, knowledge of what happened before the incident, what indeed happened and the consequences resulting will be considered. All this information helps to satisfy the requirements of Step One in the model and, for Step Two, indicates that more than one ethical maxim may be applicable.

In the first time period, before the action, two factors may be present that demand consideration: motivation and intention. What motivated the action? At times good motives produce bad results and, conversely, evil motives can produce good results. Knowledge of the motivation involved, which is not readily or easily attained, is usually a factor considered in moral reasoning. From the individual's own perspective, authenticity is a moral characteristic that applies at all times (i.e., prior to, during and following the act). Intention, the other factor, can often be discerned from the act itself, but that is not always the case. In the absence of a statement from the agent, there is no alternative, other than assessment of the act, to impute intention (Figure 3.4). This schema can also serve as a very general checklist of factors to consider when attempting to arrive at a complete description of what occurred.

Figure 3.4: Time and the Act

PRIOR TO THE ACT	DURING THE ACT	FOLLOWING THE ACT
Individual motivation and intention.	Established rules. Unwritten rules or norms.	Consequences.

Step Four—Identify and Discuss Extenuating Circumstances

At times, special or extenuating circumstances compel people to act in unusual ways. Fairness requires us to take those factors into consideration. An example, based on the sort of case reported from time to time, will provide further clarity. A young boy is admitted to the hospital with a heart defect. His pediatrician and the pediatric cardiothoracic surgeon both believe that, unless surgery is performed within a few days, the child will not survive. Even using the latest "bloodless" techniques, the surgeon is convinced a transfusion will be needed during the operation. The boy's parents, on religious grounds, object to their son receiving any blood. In response, the hospital, acting on an urgent request from the physician and surgeon, petitions the Court to make the child a ward of the Court for the duration of the treatment, so that the surgery can proceed.

Ordinarily, decisions about a child's welfare rests solely with that child's parents. By obtaining a court order, the hospital has interfered in the normal parent-child relationship. The argument presented to the Court avowed that the welfare of the boy—who would die unless the surgery was performed— represented a sufficiently strong circumstance to justify the interference. In this case, the rationale for claiming special or extenuating circumstances is both clear and strong. In many situations that is not the case at all. Serious consideration needs to be given to any factor before proposing it as a special or extenuating circumstance. Attention to this factor invokes the need, once again, for critical analysis.

Step Four is closely linked to Step One. In Step Four the facts of the case or incident are further amplified. Circumstances are best identified as extenuating or special after a full basic description of the case has been provided.

Step Five—Render Judgment

This, in one sense, is the culmination of moral reasoning. Judgment should be rendered only after all the facts, background, context and extenuating circumstances of the case have been considered and agreement reached on the ethical maxim(s) applicable.

Once we know as many of the facts as possible, and consider the special or extenuating circumstances, along with the background and context, it then becomes possible to reach a consensus among those involved in that particular moral discourse. It is not always possible to decide absolutely in terms of black or white, right or wrong, good or bad. Ethics also comes in shades of gray, that is, qualified judgments that find some right or good and some wrong or bad in a particular act. What is sought is the best decision possible based on the available knowledge, resources and a comprehensive consideration of the issues at hand. Reasons given for the judgments rendered serve as warrants to support the decision reached.

Biomedical Moral Discourse

Biomedical reflection, utilizing critical and analytical thinking and conducted within the framework of the models provided (see Chapter 5 for Model II), addresses moral dilemmas in a comprehensive, rational and just manner, taking into account diverse personal and professional beliefs. A framework is provided for reflective thinking that is both analytical and dialectical in nature. Discourse is grounded in ethical theory to provide a sound basis for moral judgments rendered.

A modicum of ethical theory has been presented and a suggested procedure, in the form of two models, has been outlined. Additional material in Chapters 4 to 6 further expand and enhance this knowledge. Elaboration of the three ethical theories (Consequential, Non-Consequential and Existentialism), presented in the next chapter, serves to strengthen the theoretical foundation of this component of medical education.

4

Sources of Ethical Decision Making

In this chapter we will explore some of the dominant sources or foundations for the contemporary ethical beliefs we may hold and act from, implicitly or explicitly. In the following sections we discuss consequentialism (teleology), non-consequentialism (deontology), and existentialism. Our purpose in presenting these three disparate views is not only to provide a balanced conceptual scenario of the realm of ethics, but also to propose a synthesis of these approaches. We provide this synthesis in order to make individual and group ethical decision making more comprehensive in an effort to establish the groundwork for a holistic understanding of biomedical ethics.

Consequentialism (Teleology): What Is Good Behavior?

Background

Consequentialism, more formally known as teleology, is an approach that argues that one must consider the ends or results of behavior rather than the intent or means used in order to render moral judgment; hence, it is situational. Within the consequential ethical orientation there exists a number of perspectives that can be classified under the headings of subjective and objective consequentialism (Macdonald and Beck-Dudley, 1994). Subjective consequentialism includes the approaches that are based upon the subjective perception of what is the best end or result to be sought; objective consequentialism or virtue ethics argues that there are basic virtues that should be adhered to, regardless of personal perception, in order to seek the best end for the individual and society. Subjective consequentialism is concerned with what should be done in a particular situation; objective consequentialism is concerned with how one should live one's life to achieve the ultimate end—happiness. Each of these orientations will be addressed in the following sections.

Subjective Consequentialism

Generally, this classification includes the ethical theories of hedonism and utilitarianism. While both are similar in the belief that the end to be sought is the greatest pleasure or good and least pain or evil, they differ in focus. This end is determined by a *test of coherence*; that is, what agrees with individual or group beliefs and desires. *Hedonism* argues that the individual should determine what is good and ethical for himself or herself by choosing whatever results in the best ratio of personal pleasure over pain. Though some hedonists argue that some pleasures are better than others (e.g., Epicurus [341-270 BC] believed that pleasures of the mind were of a higher order than pleasures of the body unlike the Cyrenaics who favored the satisfaction of desire), it remains a subjective evaluation. For example, an individual who chooses a career in the health care profession because it gives him or her financial reward, social status, the joy of scientific discovery, and/or personal emotional pleasure to treat patients can be said to be acting hedonistically.

The utilitarian focus as advocated by Jeremy Bentham (1748-1832) and J.S. Mill (1806-1873) is much more broad than that of the hedonist as it seeks the greatest pleasure and least pain for the greatest number. Determining what is the greatest pleasure continues to be a subjective calculation—a test of coherence with a belief of what is perceived to be best for the masses. Utilitarianism itself can be viewed in two distinct ways. *Act-utilitarianism* is the perspective that advocates any action that results in the greatest pleasure for the greatest number. From this view, rules, laws, policies, procedures, traditions, and individual justice can be overlooked if the results are best for the masses. For example, a researcher conducting potentially harmful experiments on patients without informed consent may attempt to justify his or her action based upon the premise that it will assist more people than it may potentially harm would be using an act-utilitarian argument.

A second form of utilitarianism advocated by the Irish philosopher Bishop George Berkeley (1687-1783) is termed *rule-utilitarianism*. Here, rules are the subject of the test—"the greatest good for the greatest number." Rules that are followed that result in the greatest good are ones that should be maintained in all circumstances; those that do not should be discarded. In contrast to the rationale provided in the previous example by the act-utilitarian, the rule-utilitarian would seek to determine if "informed consent" was a rule that would result in the greatest good. If it was perceived to do so, then, regardless of the potential outcome, breaching this rule would be unacceptable for the rule-utilitarian.

Generally, the utilitarian perspective has been more widely accepted than has hedonism as it has the tendency to promote or at least maintain some form of social awareness and responsibility. Utilitarianism is in fact the basis of not only liberal-democratic political ideology (i.e., liberalism) and economic theory (e.g., Pareto optimality), but is also the forerunner of the modern separation of ethics from religious authority. See Box A for examples of hedonism, act- and rule-utilitarianism.

The Subjective Consequential Method

The subjective consequential method has been described as the *hedonistic calculus*. It refers to a process developed by the utilitarians (i.e., Bentham) for assessing the perceived outcome of possible actions or decisions. The decision-maker is to determine the ratio of *utiles* or units of utility or pleasure for each alternative and then choose that which results in the best overall ratio of pleasure over pain. Ascertaining what would be pleasurable and painful for the masses is a function of what is perceived to cohere with the belief of the masses. For example, the utilitarian may argue that there are more units of pleasure derived by the greatest number of people by having universal health care than by privatizing health care. In contrast, the hedonist may perceive, if he or she is wealthy, that a private health care system would result in the greatest pleasure or, perhaps, the least pain for him or her.

The Advantages and Disadvantages of Subjective Consequentialism

The subjective consequentialist position has many positive aspects. First is its orientation toward the future. We do not base goodness on the past or upon tradition. Rather we base it upon what will result in the greatest future goodness. As a result, this perspective is dynamic and innovative and is capable of adapting to changing structures, medical innovation and perceptions of goodness. In a world that is changing as rapidly as ours, and with a more rapid pace of change anticipated in the twenty-first century, an ethical approach that is fluid may be essential. What was good (and possible) for us in the 1960s may not prove to be sufficient to guide us ethically in decades to come.

While flexibility and fluidity provide a dynamic ethics, subjective consequentialism may result in a weakened or unstable sense of ethical behavior. Many critics argue that the general malaise of our times is in part due to the situational nature of our ethical conduct. Where traditional ethical guidelines (or values) are no longer an explicit and stable part of our educational and societal paradigms, the resulting tendency has been an entrenchment of ruthless and self-serving behavior by individuals, organizations, communities, and nations. If ethics are dynamic, how can we establish foundations for conduct resulting in goodness? Specifically, how can we ensure that the direction of the ethical dynamic is one that fosters goodness as opposed to evil and chaos? A second advantage of subjective consequentialism is its attempt to measure goodness (i.e., the hedonistic calculus). This process fosters a rational and secular method to determine ethical conduct. Presumably, where societal and theological doctrines are diminished, ethics can enter a more detached and

Box A
Examples of Hedonism, Act-Utilitarianism and Rule-Utilitarianism in Medical Research

Hedonism. A professor and her team of researchers have received a substantial two-year grant from a pharmaceutical company to test the viability of a new drug. The company has offered to fund the project for an additional three-year period should they be satisfied with the outcome of the team's work. The professor (in search of promotion) chooses to falsify experimental data in order to ensure that subsequent research grants are received.

Act-Utilitarianism. The following examples demonstrate the disregard for the individual in favor of the perceived greatest good for the greatest number.

Researchers at the Jewish Hospital and Medical Center of Brooklyn injected live cancer cells into geriatric patients without first securing informed consent. At a New York State institution for the severely mentally challenged, children were allegedly exposed to a hepatitis virus in order to test a vaccine under controlled conditions, without adequate information being provided to parents for an informed consent. And, in Tuskegee, Alabama, black male subjects with syphilis were studied longitudinally by the U.S. Public Health Service to document the course of the untreated disease from the 1930s onwards (Kroll, 1993, p.34).

Rule-Utilitarianism. A researcher investigating the effect of minimal workloads on the functioning of a newly designed pacemaker in cardiac patients carefully follows all current experimental and ethics protocol as outlined by her nation's medical community in order to receive further funding to support her research, to enhance the financial viability of her lab and to promote the good name of her faculty and university.

scientific realm. However, can ethical issues be treated in the same manner as a hospital administrator's financial statement or a medical researcher's regression analysis? How does one assess and measure the relative merit or utility of one ethical dilemma over another?

Critics of the hedonistic calculus argue that it is difficult, indeed impossible, to quantify a concept such as *goodness*. How, for example, does one weigh the utility of one fetus over another when only one is viable in a mother's womb (see Cases 9.13 and 9.14). Furthermore, is it possible for the decision-maker to forecast accurately the consequence of his or her action? Can the decision-maker ever exhaust all possible alternatives without incurring decision paralysis? Finally, does one know, in fact, what is *good*? How well does the decision-maker's perception cohere with that of the greatest number? Does the decision-maker's subjective perception of coherence not destroy the supposed scientific basis of this method? Is it possible to determine a consensus at all regarding what is *good*?

Subjective consequentialism, in its utilitarian form, provides an explicit concern for the welfare of the masses. Its dictum "the greatest good for the greatest number" is testimony to the decision-maker's obligation to the populace as opposed to personal survival. However, can we warrant forsaking the minority's or the individual's rights to serve the majority's will? For example, should we prevent the transplant of vital organs to individuals with Down's Syndrome because they are less functional or productive members of society? Can we condone the actions of health care administrators who close rural hospitals in favor of cost-benefit ratios and the general efficient operations of the health care system despite the real possibility that some individual patients may suffer as a result? Yet, fundamental to utilitarianism is faith in the collective will being just to the greatest number.

Can we be sure that this collective wisdom satisfies our perception or our intuitive belief in what is ethical conduct? Further, can we be so certain of the actual coherence of the wisdom of the collective? The populace can be notoriously wrong, superficial, uniformed and inconsistent. To see that collective wisdom and common sense can be erroneous, one needs only to recall such historical examples as the letting of blood for various ills, the firm belief that "evil" was the cause of the Black Plague of the medieval era, and the jailing of Copernicus for suggesting that the earth orbited the sun.

Objective Consequentialism

Objective consequentialism or virtue ethics is usually associated with the traditional teleological perspective advocated by Aristotle (384-322 BC) in his treatise entitled *Nichomachean Ethics*. Where subjective consequentialism relies on the test of coherence, that is, coheres with other perceptions or beliefs, objective consequentialism is based upon the *test of correspondence*. This view, it is argued, corresponds with what is believed to be objectively true of human nature and human potentiality. As a result, it is less a preference or emotional desire than a standard that any human as a human ought to follow because it corresponds with what it is to be a fulfilled human.

According to Aristotle, human behavior is end-driven (i.e., teleological). As the end of the health care profession is the general health of the population, the ultimate end of all human endeavor is happiness or *eudaimonia*. Happiness, in this sense, is not the happiness one may feel when receiving a raise in pay or completing nursing or medical school or falling in love. Rather happiness is the end point of all of one's efforts to flourish as a human. In other words, one seeks happiness as the ultimate end of a life well lived. To flourish as a human, Aristotle believes that one must live virtuously (and have good luck). To live virtuously is to habitually base one's actions upon virtues such as courage, wisdom, temperance, and justice. Each virtue is a mean between deficiency and excess. For example, courage is the mean between cowardice and recklessness; generosity is the mean between stinginess and extravagance. Virtues are particular or natural to humans and distinguish us from non-rational animals—they make us uniquely human. Aristotle argues that

> Neither by nature ... nor contrary to nature do the virtues arise in us; rather we are adapted to receive them, and are made perfect by habit.... [T]he virtues we get by first exercising them, as also happens in the case of the arts as well. For the things we have to learn before we can do them, e.g., men become builders by building and lyre players by playing the lyre; so too we become just by doing just acts, temperate by doing temperate acts, brave by doing brave acts (1968, p.952).

We have the ability though to choose not to actualize and habitualize these virtues; that is, to make decisions that are not in accordance with virtue. Consequently, it is possible not to lead fulfilled or virtuous lives and thus fail to achieve true happiness or *eudaimonia* (as opposed to apparent happiness). However, if we are able to distinguish between excess and deficit and choose the mean between these extremes, then, presumably, virtuous behavior and happiness are within our grasp.

While this approach may appear to be highly individualistic, it must be noted that Aristotle believed that virtuous behavior (and, in particular, just behavior) ultimately led to a just and happy society. The virtuous individual was considered the essential building block for the good society. This is in contrast with the utilitarian focus upon the "greatest good for the greatest number" and its obfuscation of the individual.

Aristotle would argue that virtuous health care professionals would exhibit these virtues not only in their professional lives but also in their private lives in order to achieve happiness or a fulfilled life as a human. As happiness is the "activity of the soul in accordance with virtue," any behavior, professional or personal, that is not virtuous essentially damages the soul and thus inhibits the individual from achieving *eudaimonia*.

The Objective Consequential Method

Objective consequentialism is an ethical theory of choice and of habit. The decision-maker has the capacity to choose behavior that is in accordance with virtue as well as to reject, ignore, or remain ignorant of virtue. Objective consequentialism is an experiential ethical theory. Aristotle argues that the decision-maker must experience virtuous behavior in order to be virtuous. One must act prudently to be prudent, and act generously to be generous, courageously to be courageous. Further, in order to realize eudaimonia, virtuous behavior must become habitual. One virtuous act does not make a virtuous person. Thus, the decision-maker must become well grounded in choosing the "golden mean" between extremes and have this become second nature in order to live virtuously.

The Advantages and Disadvantages of Objective Consequentialism

One clear advantage of this school of thought is that it focuses not upon a particular incident (i.e., I am faced with an ethical dilemma, what should I do now?) but upon an ethical life well-lived. It encourages life-long ethical or virtuous conduct rather than a concern for ethics when occasion demands.

This method can lead, however, to some ambiguity regarding what is accepted as a virtue (e.g., varying perceptions based upon cultural differences), how this virtue is to be interpreted into my particular context (e.g., as a physician or nurse), and how one might deal with circumstances that call for the resolution between conflicting virtues. For example, if a spouse is informed that her husband is terminally ill and she emphatically argues that her husband's current mental state is too fragile to accept such information, a physician is faced with the conflict between the virtues of honesty and prudence. To which virtue does one appeal?

Non-Consequentialism (Deontology): What Is Right Behavior?

Background

Non-consequentialism, also identified as formalism or deontology, is an approach that considers the means, principles or personal duties as the foundation for "right" ethical conduct. This perspective is in obvious contrast with consequentialism, as the ends of action or decision making become secondary to the formal adherence to rule-based behavior. The basis or grounding of non-consequentialism varies and includes *theology, social contract* and *intuition* orientations.

Theology. Religious doctrine is the basis of a theological orientation. The Bible, the Koran, and the Bhagavad Gita provide us with three examples of publications that contain theologically based principles of ethical conduct. As followers of any one of these or other possible religious teachings, it is the sacred duty of the believer to abide by the words of God or the gods. Thus, we measure one's behavior against established religious doctrine or rule. For example, the Ten Commandments and the Old Testament give clear direction for the ethical conduct of the Christian and Jew. The more orthodox a person's religious beliefs, it appears, the more sacrosanct is the literal interpretation of the doctrine, and, arguably, the less room for individual interpretation.

Social Contract. A second orientation of this approach argues for a secular set of rules. One must obey these rules, not only to make life better as a member of a collective, but also to avoid the persecution of the populace. The social contract made, both implicitly and explicitly, by all members of society establishes the parameters of acceptable and preferred "right" conduct. This contract is manifested in macro-perspectives through the laws governing society-at-large, as well as in micro-perspectives through those policies and procedures that form the basis for right conduct in our institutional life.

Why is it necessary, for example, to formalize rules of conduct in the workplace or on the tennis court? Generally we do so to enhance the quality of life for each individual. Hobbes has suggested that life without society (and rules/laws) is "nasty, brutish, and short." Aristotle argues that we are social or political animals. Achieving the "good life" that we all seek is, therefore, impossible without being a part of the collective; we cannot realize or express virtuous behavior alone. Rousseau (1979) says that

> although in civil society man surrenders some of the advantages that belong to a state of nature [i.e., a state of complete individual freedom], he gains in return greater ones.... Man acquires with civil society, moral freedom, which alone makes man the master of himself; for to be governed by appetite alone is slavery, while obedience to a law one prescribes to oneself is freedom (p.65).

For example, in organized sport, we enter competition based upon a mutually accepted code of conduct (i.e., the rules). This code is not heaven sent nor is it necessarily the result of intuitive guidance. Individuals (sometimes generations of individuals) interested in playing a game in a particular manner create and agree upon the code or rules of the game. We play eighteen holes of golf rather than twelve because of a historical social contract among early Scottish enthusiasts. Clearly, social conventions and mores become central to this orientation.

Intuition. A third view argues in favor of an intuitive approach. Intuition, in this context, is not considered as a hunch or a gut reaction. We can logically defend intuition as it refers to a reasoned process. Perhaps the most famous proponent of this view is Immanuel Kant. He suggested that a profound commonality among all humans is the capacity to reason. Through this generic capacity, we are capable of coming to terms with universal notions of right, duty and self-evident ethical conduct. According to Kant (1968), in what he formally termed the categorical imperative, we find the criterion for establishing right behavior. This imperative states that one ought to "act only according to that maxim by which you can at the same time will that it should become a universal law" (p.45). We, therefore, perceive such an act as ethically valid for all and for all time. One cannot lie, cheat or steal unless one could argue that everyone ought to lie, cheat and steal.

The essential feature, then, of non-consequentialism is doing one's duty. This duty is placed upon us from religious sources, from societal contracts or from our innate and self-evident capacity to reason. To place this perspective in context, the following example (Box B) describes the non-consequentialist behavior of a hospital administrator.

Justice. Theories of justice are, broadly speaking, non-consequential or deontological in nature as they are fundamentally rule-based. However, these theories generally provide much more prescriptive guidance for the decision-maker than does Kant's categorical imperative. Perhaps the two best-known positions come to us from both ancient and contemporary sources.

The notion of justice has a long philosophical tradition dating back to the Socratic era. Aristotle paid considerable attention to it in his *Nichomachean Ethics* in which he stated that "[j]ustice ... is not a part of virtue but the whole of virtue; its opposite, unjustice, is not part of vice but the whole of vice" (1971, p.157). Aristotle distinguishes between distributive and rectificatory or corrective justice. Distributive justice refers to the principle which states that equals ought to be treated equally and unequals ought to be treated unequally (i.e., justice is proportionate). Rectificatory justice refers to the principle which suggests that inequalities ought to be restored to form just proportions.

Rawls (1971) provides a contemporary perspective of justice. His theory is concerned primarily with the notion of social justice and the means to obtain maximization of rewards for the disadvantaged. His approach begins with the introduction of the ideal observer who, under a "veil of ignorance," must develop principles of justice in a society where one cannot know one's station in life (i.e., advantaged or disadvantaged, Catholic or Buddhist, male or female). Rawls proposes that each person will be bound to the principles formulated

> in future circumstances the peculiarities of which cannot be known and which might well be such that the principle is then to his disadvantage.... The principles will express the conditions in accordance with which each person is the least unwilling to have his interests limited in the design of practices, given the competing interests of the others, on the supposition that the interests of the others will be limited likewise (pp.373-374).

Box B
An Example of Non-Consequentialism in Hospital Administration

A new administrator in an urban and severely understaffed hospital is made aware that at least two of her nurses are in the habit of taking "uppers" while on long shifts and use alcohol occasionally prior to commencing work. The source of this information is the spouse of an intern who is concerned that her husband is going to be blamed eventually for the negligence of the nurses in the Operating Room. She is threatening to "whistle blow" if nothing is done about the issue. The administrator was unaware of any drug culture among the hospital's staff.

As an individual whose ethical basis is non-consequentialism, she may pursue this dilemma in the following manner: First, determine if the behavior of the staff can pass the test of categorical imperative. Could their behavior be accepted as universally right? If not, then she must determine what is her duty as the person responsible for the actions of staff. She may again appeal to the categorical imperative to establish what maxim of professional duty should be employed; that is, what rule would be universally valid. In conjunction with this, she may also turn to her legal responsibility as well as established principles of administrative and staff behavior (e.g., code of ethics) to determine what society and the profession have deemed a priori ethical.

In this sense, the administrator has considered her duty from cosmopolitan, societal, and organizational deontological or non-consequential perspectives. [N.B., For a more indepth discussion of cosmopolitan, local, and individual locus of analysis in non-profit organizations, see Agarwal, J. & Malloy, D.C. (1998), Ethical work climate dimensions in a non-profit organization: An empirical investigation, Journal of Business Ethics, 17.] The result of each of these levels of inquiry most likely points toward the immediate cessation of this behavior as it contravenes universally accepted behavior, Canadian law, and hospital policy.

The result of this deductive process, according to Rawls, is the formulation of two principles—the liberty principle and the difference principle. The liberty principle refers to the equal access for all persons to such basic human liberties as freedom of speech and religion, and freedom to own property. The second principle provides the conditions allowing the first principle to be overridden. That is, inequality can be accepted when the advantages of all persons is the result of the transgression of the liberty principle. For example, a physician has the power to write prescriptions for patients. This unique role of the physician is a safeguard against the layperson from acquiring drugs at will (i.e., the liberty principle) that may be harmful to individuals and the public if abused. This manifestation of the difference principle (i.e., the power to write prescriptions) is accepted by the general population as a necessary condition to override its liberty and thus enhances its general welfare.

Rawls suggests that individuals acting in their own self-interest will generally place emphasis upon the principle of liberty and then agree to the allowable departures from it. In other words, the individual will choose to err on the side of one's own advantage. Rawl's theory of justice has particular relevance for the administrative aspect of the health care profession. Policies, procedures, and organizational hierarchies exist by definition in bureaucracies and will inevitably create many inequities.

The Non-Consequential Method

Unlike the hedonistic calculus of the utilitarians, the non-consequentialists do not employ a cost-benefit analysis or an explicit formula to determine ethical worth. Rather, the decision-maker is to refer to his or her intuitive and rational sense of what would be universally right. This perspective represents a cognitive logic by which truth and rightness become self-evident for all rational people. Or, the decision-maker may appeal to sets of rules, codes, and principles established by religious or secular sources (i.e., societal, cultural, or organizational) (Hodgkinson, 1996).

The Advantages and Disadvantages of Non-Consequentialism

The primary advantage of this approach is that it considers the manner and intent of our actions as opposed to simply allowing the ends to justify the means. This is in contrast, as we discovered, with most forms of consequentialism. Non-consequentialism does not allow for the (teleological) suspension of what we instinctively reason to be just in order to achieve the best end. As a result, it can be argued, there is an appeal to our intuitive sense of rightness.

In addition, the notion of duty is a central feature of this view. As religion and society play a key role in this theory, traditional precepts and obligations represent significant criteria against which behavior is judged. We look to what tradition tells us is right. The impact of this formalism is stability in cultural ethical expectations.

The elements that point to the strengths of non-consequentialism also expose its inherent weaknesses. As rules and principles are the frameworks for ethical judgment, the individual's personal responsibility for ethical conduct is deferred to externally driven criteria (e.g., religion or society is to praise or to blame). For example, Adolph Eichmann, the architect of the slaughter of Jews in World War II, attempted to argue his innocence by suggesting that he was merely following orders (organizational principles). The problem is that some principles are eventually deemed to be unjust. An example of this was Martin Luther King, who argued from his jail cell that it is every person's responsibility to abide by just laws, yet, at the same time, we must reject those that are unjust (i.e., segregation).

Further, the reality of societal change places enormous pressure upon the validity, and perhaps the reliability, of traditional notions of ethical conduct. For example, just a few decades ago a competitive "market" for human organ transplantation did not exist. The medical profession was not faced with the overwhelming decision to give or not to give a patient a life-sustaining organ based upon the patient's age or health practices (i.e., alcohol, tobacco, or other drug abuse). This is certainly a reality today. These and similar circumstances brought about by developments in science and in society place new pressure upon traditional notions and interpretations of what is the right thing to do.

Where consequentialism's dynamics provide for flexibility as society changes, non-consequentialism's static nature may hinder it from providing a contemporary basis from which to judge rightness and wrongness. As a result, traditional notions of ethics may become static, dead, irrelevant and ignored.

Having briefly surveyed the ends and means approaches to ethical behavior, the reader may wonder which way to turn to determine what, in fact, is moral behavior? One possible answer can be found in the next approach which is a radical departure from consequentialism and non-consequentialism. Existentialism has been termed a revolt against traditional philosophy and argues for a paradigmatically different approach to ethical conduct compared to the former two theories.

Existentialism: What Is Authentic Behavior?

Background

Existentialism is a disjointed school of thought. It consists of a disparate and eclectic set of ideas gathered from a dissimilar group of philosophical thinkers. While existentialists, as individual thinkers, differ dramatically, two common threads of thought are woven throughout their ideas regarding the nature of ethical conduct. The first is the belief in the freedom of individuals to create their own essence, that is, to create who they are. Sartre, a twentieth century French existentialist, argued that "existence precedes essence." This implies that we exist as humans, and we then become whom we decide to be through our free will or choice. We are not predetermined. Who we are is not purely the result of either societal reinforcement (nurture) or our genetic predisposition (nature). Existentialists would suggest that, through our capacity to exercise free will, we are the sums of the decisions made through that capacity.

The second component of existentialism is contained in the concept of responsibility for one's actions. What has been labeled the "terrible freedom," the "agony of thinking" or the "torment of choice" posits the responsibility for correct behavior squarely on the shoulders of the individual. That one is responsible for all of one's actions and the impact of these actions upon all of humanity is cause for the alleged fear and despair that the existentialist experiences as one's essence is created. As a result, behavior, "good" or "right," "bad" or "wrong," cannot be diverted to an external locus of control. For example, an individual ought not to praise or blame co-workers, policy, clients, patients or society for the success or failure of his or her acts. Further, this individual cannot argue that responsibility will be taken for personal acts only. All action must be considered as it may influence all individuals, all of society or all of humanity.

Though this theory is highly personal, it is not about selfishness nor is it hedonistic. Rather, existentialism is a philosophy that insists that the individual is self-determined and must constantly battle to overcome the "averaging" effect of modern society. It acknowledges respect for individualism, yet acknowledges the tremendous responsibility that one's individualism and its accompanying decisions have for others. For example, the great existentialist Sartre (1997) suggests that

> When we say that man chooses himself, we do not mean that every one of us must choose himself; but by that we also mean that in choosing for himself he chooses for all men.... What we choose is always the better and nothing can be better unless it is better for all.... Our responsibility is thus much greater than we had supposed, for it concerns mankind as a whole (p.586).

Thus, it is blatantly a misinterpretation to suggest that existentialism is glorified hedonism. An example of existential thinking in a medical context is provided below (see Box C).

The Existential Method

The method for the existentialist consists of one criterion—authenticity. All action must be judged against the individual's genuineness. To be authentic or genuine implies being honest with oneself and with others. Shakespeare's

Box C
An Example of Existentialism in Medicine

Mr. and Mrs. M. were an elderly couple in their eighties. Mrs. M. had recently fallen and broken her clavicle and her left tibia. As a result, she was unable to care for herself and the tasks of dressing, bathing and feeding Mrs. M. fell upon her husband. He was happy to take this on despite his own limited capacities. As luck would have it, Mr. M. slipped and fell in front of the grocery store and broke his hip. Both Mr. and Mrs. M. had to be admitted to an elderly care unit while they both recuperated from their injuries. Upon arriving at the care facility, the couple was informed that in addition to the medication they were taking for pain, they would be given sleeping pills nightly. Both Mr. and Mrs. M. refused, as they were somewhat adverse to taking any medication at all and worried that their mental capacities would be permanently hampered as a consequence.

Sue was the night nurse. She was a recent graduate working at her first position. She was very enthusiastic and felt that she had a very bright career ahead. Sue read the chart for Mr. M.'s medication that was written earlier in the evening by the attending physician. A mild dose of sleeping pills was prescribed. Sue proceeded to Mr. M.'s room and informed him of the nature of his evening medication—which he summarily refused to take. She returned to the nursing station and expressed to the other nurses her concern and frustration with Mr. M. The head nurse was part of this conversation and instructed Sue that it was imperative that he take his medication—it was "doctor's orders." It was suggested that she tell the patient that he didn't have to take the green pills but the pink pills were vitamin supplements and that they would have no effect on him (they were, in fact, sleeping pills). Sue proceeded down the hall and before entering Mr. M.'s room the magnitude of the situation hit her full force—Do I reject the patient's right to informed consent by lying to him about his medication, or do I follow the explicit orders of this patient's physician and the head nurse (who essentially held Sue's career in her hands)?

Sue, now in conflict between patient and medical staff and between the principles of informed consent and duty to her superiors, had to decide what to do and quickly—the "agony of choice" was intimately being experienced: (1) the patient was clear in his preference, (2) the head nurse was clear in her orders and those of the physician, (3) Sue was deeply committed to patients' rights. Sue decided to reject the deception suggested by the head nurse and the written orders of the physician. She was determined to make Mr. M. aware of the options and consequences of taking or rejecting the medication and then to have him choose (i.e., informed consent). She was prepared to take full responsibility for her actions which she knew were authentic for her and the correct decision for Mr. M. and for all patients. In this way, Sue was functioning fully as Sartre would expect her to do as an existentialist. Her decision was indeed hers and she chose to maintain her own authenticity. Yet, at the same time, Sue chose for all patients, and she was prepared to take responsibility for her actions and suffer the wrath of the head nurse and the implication for her career.

dictum "To thyne own self be true" is an appropriate metaphor for the existential method. As we have mentioned, this is perhaps the most difficult approach as there is no method, no formula, no rule, principle or maxim to help in choosing a course of action. The existentialist will never have more than his or her authenticity and therefore will always experience the "agony of choice." As a person comes to accept "nothingness" (i.e., the constant state of becoming who they are), it is then possible to deal more readily with the solitude and responsibility of individual decision-making behavior. While this method may appear to be a non-method, that is, in fact, the existentialist's lot.

The Advantages and Disadvantages of Existentialism

Existentialism is one of the most demanding theories of ethical conduct. This is because the full weight of individual action rests upon the decision-maker. All choices must be made from within the soul or the will of the individual, as opposed to following externally driven, rational, cost-benefit analyses (consequentialism) or principles (non-consequentialism). This is the central advantage of existentialism, as it leads to complete honesty with oneself and with all others who may be influenced by one's actions.

The foremost disadvantage of existentialism is that it does not provide a clear means to deciding one's essence or authenticity. The individual is left entirely alone in deciding which is the best choice. No God, process or societal norm can make the choice for the individual. Some may believe that this theory is too depressing, since existentialism argues that there is no meaning to the universe, that God is dead and that we are essentially alone and nothing. This, however, has its optimistic side as well. That we are nothing also implies that we are capable of becoming. Individuals are completely free and unfettered to create whom, in fact, they wish to be if there is no God and no predestination and if society does not hold all the answers.

We have now discussed the essence of three very different approaches to ethical thought. In the following section, a composite of these views is provided, based upon the premise that this step will give the reader a more comprehensive perspective of ethical action and decision making.

Synthesis: Good, Right and Authentic Behavior

Thus far we have discussed three disparate approaches that identify the good, the right and the authentic aspects of ethical behavior. Taken individually, we have observed that each presents a particular view of what constitutes ethical conduct. On the other hand, each individually provides an incomplete perspective. Consequentialism identifies the good and dynamic change while neglecting the right and the authentic. Non-consequentialism considers the right and the stable (i.e., the traditional notions of right) yet overlooks the good and the authentic. Finally, existentialist thought views authenticity as primary, while perhaps obfuscating the good and the right. If each presents an incomplete picture, can there be an acceptable synthesis to create good, right and authentic behavior? Is there a holistic behavior that meets all the criteria?

We argue that it is possible and preferable that individuals, when confronted with an ethical dilemma, incorporate criteria from each of these theories to form a complete ethical decision. This synthesis may be analogous to the ancient Roman God of the Gates. This god possessed two faces, which enabled him to look inwards to protect the people within the city and outwards to protect them from invaders. Our synthesis has this Janus-head, with three faces instead of two. One face looks toward the future, the dynamic and the good. Another looks backwards to the past, the stable and the right. Finally, one faces inward, at the essence, the freedom, the responsibility and the authenticity of the individual.

Complete ethical decisions may be formulated within the following framework:

1. Does the decision accomplish the best end for the greatest number?

2. Is the decision consistent with intuitive, organizational, socio-cultural and universal norms?

3. Is this free, honest and authentic behavior? How does this particular decision impact on oneself? And on others who will feel the impact?

A decision based upon these criteria, then, can presumably be considered ethically complete—good, right and authentic. That is, such a decision will accomplish the goal (the good), it will do so based upon inclusive means (the right), and it will be reflective of the decision-maker's authentic intent.

We argue that the synthesis of good, right and authentic decision making is comprehensive. A decision that is not based upon these criteria, we suggest, cannot be considered ethically complete and must be re-evaluated; another alternative must be found. The search for this synthesis requires a great deal of contemplation. Such inquiry and introspection is difficult. Though the world of medicine is characterized by its fast pace, when it comes to ethical behavior, we may wish to accept the notion that the person who does not hesitate (and reflect) may be lost.

In this chapter we have briefly surveyed the consequential, non-consequential, and existential schools of ethical thought. While each theory argues for different criteria to judge ideal conduct, each provides us with an incomplete perspective. In response to this fragmented picture have we provided the reader with a model in which the synthesis of the good, the right and the authentic nature of complete ethical decisions is contained. In the next chapter, we will explore the many moderators that may influence, to a greater or lesser extent, the decision-making behavior of the individual.

5

Moderators Influencing Ethical Decision Making

A s you have probably gathered from the preceding chapters, ethics is a rather complicated yet fascinating field of practical living and academic study. By now you have discovered that to say that an act is ethical or unethical can be too simplistic a statement. Having read thus far, you are aware that detecting the ethical disposition of an act requires complex patterns of analysis and thought, along with rigor in the application of moral reasoning. In this chapter and the next, we present our second model of ethical decision making (Figure 5.1).

Model II—A Comprehensive Approach

This model provides the reader with a more comprehensive approach to resolving moral dilemmas because it identifies a variety of moderators or variables that may, to a greater or lesser extent, influence the manner in which one makes ethical decisions. A significant aspect of this model is that it can be used, not only to render judgment of past events (as is the case with our first model), but it can also enable the decision-maker to assess comprehensively future courses of ethical conduct. We believe that by adopting this model, not only in the cases presented in Chapter 9, but also in actual day-to-day dilemmas, you will enhance the rigor, reduce the ambiguity and increase the effectiveness of your ethical reasoning.

The manner in which we make decisions, ethical or unethical, is most often the result of a multitude of moderators. These moderators are shown in Figure 5.1. If we are to understand why individuals behave in the way they do, it is necessary to investigate some antecedent features. These features may, based on the individual's level of moral reasoning or psychological development, influence behavior. We have chosen to categorize these variables into five sets of moderators. The first set concerns those moderators that are particular to the individual. They include such variables as ethical and value grounding, level of moral development and demographic moderators, such as age, education and gender.

Figure 5-1: Ethical Decision Making Model—Comprehensive Approach

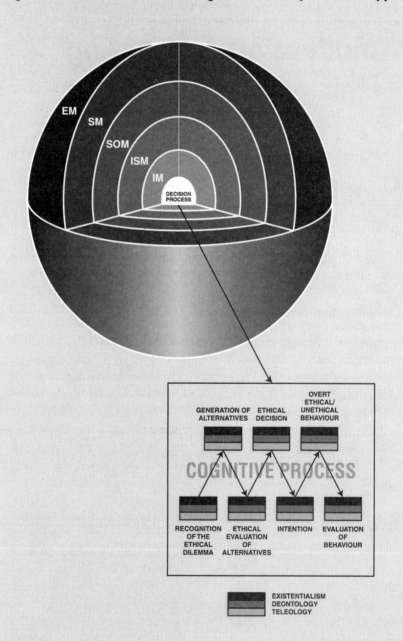

The second set contains moderators that involve the relationships that the decision-maker has with significant others. These relationships include those with family and friends, peers, group members, individuals from other communities and organizations. The nature of the ethical dilemma itself is a third area that we consider to be a potential influence on ethical behavior. The fourth set of moderators considers the organizational or team culture in which an individual is participating, working or volunteering. The final category includes moderators that are external to the individual and organizational context. These moderators include political, social, economic and technical variables that may influence the manner in which decisions are made, of an ethical or unethical nature. In the following paragraphs, each area will be explored in detail.

I. Individual Moderators of Ethical Decision Making

In this section we describe the effect that an individual's ethical orientation, level of moral development, and demographic profile may have upon decision-making behavior.

1. Ethical Orientation. Ethical orientation forms the basis of the content of our behavior. Awareness of our ethical nature tells us to what extent we focus upon good, right and authentic behavior and what is bad, wrong and inauthentic. If our nature is to behave as a teleologist, the content of our behavior may be predisposed to seeking out the good ends in decision making. If, on the other hand, we tend to be more deontological in our behavior, the means become the dominant concern. For example, the teleologist's theme could be "to succeed at all cost," whereas the deontologist's theme could be "it is not to win or lose but how one plays the game."

In contrast to these dispositions is the existential view, which places all weight upon freedom, responsibility and authenticity. The ends and the means pale in comparison to the importance of exercising freedom and one's own creative will. The existentialist theme is, as expressed so directly by Nietzsche, "Do something! Exist!"

Though we have identified, here and in earlier chapters, three extreme positions or archetypes, it is important to realize that few of us represent or exhibit pure forms of any one orientation. Research informs us that we are hybrids of all of these ethical positions and that our orientation is often contextually driven; it is an eclectic mix (e.g., Reidenbach and Robin, 1988, 1990).

Once identified, we must then decide if that ethical orientation is how we want to continue believing and behaving. Does my action follow my beliefs and values? Do I, for example, profess the existential axiom of freedom yet seldom take responsibility for my action, or do I spread the blame on those around me? Similarly, can we identify the behavior of our co-workers and

peers as focused upon the ends or the means? Are we aware of their commitment to their own authenticity? For example, can we conclude from our
observation of an individual's behavior that there is a propensity toward goal
accomplishment, rule following or genuineness?

Ethical orientation influences how we behave. The schools of ethics that
we have covered provide us with tools with which we can describe our own
behavior and that of those around us. As a result, we have a clearer idea of
what we and those around do that is ethically good, right and authentic.

2. Cognitive Moral Development. From a different perspective, researchers
in cognitive moral development have sought to explain moral behavior in
terms of the level of the individual's cognitive complexity. Following Piaget's
work studying the moral development of children, the research conducted by
Laurence Kohlberg and his colleagues in the 1970's and 80's as well as
research that continues today employing Kohlberg's model and method, particularly in the area of applied ethics (e.g., business and administrative ethics),
has examined the rationale for moral behavior among adolescents and adults.
While Kohlberg's work has received substantial support, there are critics who
have argued against his methodology and his theoretical assumptions. These
criticisms were initially raised by Carol Gilligan who argued that the Kohlber-
gian model was biased against women. Her approach, which she termed the
Ethics of Care, attempted to provide a feminine alternative to the so-called
masculine model. In the following sections each of these perspectives will be
discussed. [**N.B.,** It should be noted that much of the debate between these two
perspectives is based upon vying theoretical and empirical assumptions. We
will not explore this debate and would recommend the following text as a
good resource to explore the Kohlberg-Gilligan dialectic: Shogun, D. (1988),
Care and Moral Motivation, Toronto, Ontario, OISE Press.]

Kohlberg's Model. This model, developed from the responses of subjects to
hypothetical moral dilemmas, is structured in three levels consisting of two
stages per level. These levels are termed *pre-conventional, conventional,* and
post-conventional. The *pre-conventional* level is characterized by reasoning
focused upon the individual's own survival. It is a hedonistic orientation. At
this level, pain is avoided and reward, as exchange, is sought. Behavior at this
level is, therefore, not a function of lofty principles or concern for others.
Rather, this level is egocentric and selfish. A pre-conventional employee is
likely to strive to gain extrinsic rewards (e.g., money) or to avoid punishment
(e.g., fear of physical, verbal or monetary reprisals for poor performance).

The *conventional* level describes reasoning focused upon one's significant
others and society-at-large. At this level, behavior is not self-centered; rather it
is based upon the approval one seeks from those with whom one has close
interpersonal relationships or from the greater community. Seeking the approval of the patient, fellow nurses and physicians, hospital administrators, or

the public may drive the conventional individual to act in a particular manner. Individuals who reason from either the conventional or pre-conventional levels are externally driven. In other words, the rationale for their behavior is based upon sources external to themselves.

Individuals whose reasoning is complex and based upon their personal commitment to the medical profession specifically and to universal principles of justice generally would be considered by Kohlberg to be post-conventional in their cognitive moral development. These people reason not from selfishness, nor do they necessarily reason from the influence of the collective will of those around them. Rather, because of their own introspection, intelligence, moral advancement and maturity, they have come to reason in complex and highly personal ways toward resolutions they hold as right, good and authentic modes of behavior.

The proponents of this post-conventional approach argue that the way in which an individual can achieve more complex levels of moral reasoning is primarily through an environment that is progressively enriching. This environment, whether it is enriching educationally or experientially, provides opportunities for individuals to have their cognitive schema (i.e., the conceptual maps we have created to explain the world around us) challenged, critiqued and broadened. Because of such challenges to our worldview, we may rethink our positions and opt for a more complex explanation of reality. What we understand, in other words, does not simply align in dichotomies of black or white, right or wrong, good or bad, but is a result of many cognitive and affective "shades of grey."

The Ethic of Caring. Carol Gilligan (1982), a colleague of Kohlberg's at Harvard, believed that another cognitive approach was needed that would explain more accurately the manner in which females reason morally. Using open-ended interviews with female subjects, she found that the underlying rationale for the behavior of females was the notion of relationship and *caring* as opposed to justice. Her model consists of three levels and two transitional phases.

The first level is similar to Kohlberg's pre-conventional level as it is fundamentally self-centred and focused upon personal survival. Here, one cares only for oneself. This level is followed by the first transition in which the female begins to recognize that there are other individuals to whom she is responsible. In this stage, the female begins to break out of her ego-centric perspective and starts to realize additional obligations and attachments to others. This transition is followed by the second level in which the female becomes altruistic in her concern for others at the expense of her own moral care. She is not only aware of her relations and responsibilities to others, she also believes that she must care for all of these individuals and becomes the *selfless mother* figure that Gilligan argues is a function of societal expectation as opposed to the truth (i.e., that altruism is not necessarily the same as goodness). This level leads to a second transition in which the women recognizes that truth is not altruism and that she herself is in need of care and control. The final stage of Gilligan's model describes the morality of nonviolence or caring. Here the woman has rejected the traditional criterion of feminine morality (i.e., self-abnegation and self-sacrifice) in favor of one in which care becomes the universal obligation where "the worth of the self in relation to others, the claiming of the power to choose, and the acceptance of responsibility for choice" (p.507) now becomes the paramount issue. The woman now becomes

> the arbiter of an independent judgment that now subsumes both conventions and individual needs under the moral principle of nonviolence. Judgment remains psychological in its concern with the intention and consequence of action, but now it becomes universal in its condemnation of exploitation and hurt (p.492).

The work of Gilligan first revealed the unique feminine character of moral development (morality of caring). The implications of her research are significant particularly if the notion of moral development (i.e., Kohlberg's model) is conceptually inaccurate for the female population. Acknowledging the inherent differences in moral reasoning between genders may enhance the practitioner's ability to explain and understand ethical or unethical behavior.

The juxtaposition of Kohlberg and Gilligan are of special interest in the health care profession as both the ethic of justice and the ethic of caring models resonate loudly in medical decision making. Ensuring that physicians and nurses adhere to established policies and practices is fundamental to patient health and safety, as well as the efficient and effective operation of any health care unit. On the other hand, the health care profession is more than abiding by rules and regulations and repairing damaged subjects. It includes the holistic well-being of the patient and fellow professionals (e.g., the Hippocratic oath). For example, the health care professional should consider the cardiac patient as an individual with fears, concerns, and family and friends who worry and need emotional care as opposed to simply a body with a dysfunctional heart in need of technical intervention.

The value of using an approach based upon cognitive moral development is two-fold. First, it provides a framework from which we may better understand the rationale for our own behavior and that of the individuals with whom we interact. Unlike ethics, which tells us the content or substance of behavior, cognitive developmental psychology explains why we make decisions the way we do. For example, do we abide by the law because of a pre-conventional fear of avoiding punishment or is it a post-conventional personal commitment to justice? A schematic representation of this framework is provided in Figure 5.2.

Figure 5.2: Kohlberg's (1969) Model of Moral Development

Level I—Pre-Conventional Morality

Stage 1	Punishment orientation	Obeys rules to avoid punishment.
Stage 2	Reward orientation	Conforms to obtain rewards, to have favors returned.

Level II—Conventional Morality

Stage 3	Good boy/girl orientation	Conforms to avoid disapproval of others.
Stage 4	Authority orientation	Blindly accepts social conventions and rules (i.e., law and order morality).

Level III—Post-Conventional Morality

Stage 5	Social contract orientation	Conforms to Hobbesian and Lockian contract theory. One's duty is to avoid violating contractual or natural rights.
Stage 6	Ethical principle orientation	Actions guided by self-chosen ethical principles.

3. Demographic Profile. Demography refers to the variety of background moderators, such as age, education, sex, race or ethnicity, cultural background, place of residence, among many other variables. Each of these variables may have a profound influence on the way in which individuals act and perceive ethical and unethical conduct. The research in this area is, however, rather mixed.

While there is some trend toward more enhanced ethical perception and behavior among older and more educated subjects, there is less consensus when gender and sexuality differences are measured. Whether females and males reason differently about ethical issues and whether they employ different ethical criteria is far from conclusive.

From another perspective, cross-cultural research has demonstrated that significant differences exist in the way in which members of different cultures reason ethically. This is not to say, however, that any one ethnic culture portrays "superior" ethical reasoning or behavior. Suffice it to say that each of us brings a unique essence that may influence, to a greater or lesser extent, the manner in which ethical conduct is perceived and acted upon. It is up to us as unique individuals to recognize that our behavior forms and informs our own essence and to accept the consequences of, and responsibility for, all of our actions. Further, once one recognizes the positive and negative aspects of one's demographic profile, the decision to change or maintain one's ethical position can be made.

II. Significant Other Moderators of Ethical Decision Making

These moderators include interpersonal, inter-organizational, and extra-organizational relationships that an individual has with other potentially influential persons. Interpersonal relationships are those special connections we have with family, friends, co-workers and mentors. These persons may play a significant part in the development of our initial moral character.

These persons are the ones who perhaps initially taught us all the values we now unquestioningly hold. For many, behavior is based upon seeking approval from these significant others. As a result, the influence of these significant others upon our perceptions and behavior can be powerful.

A second grouping of relationships may also provide a strong incentive to behave ethically or unethically. Much research has been conducted into the impact of a co-worker's behavior and, more important, a supervisor's behavior upon the individual. Supervisors are particularly relevant because they, as leaders, are perceived by many as role models and representatives of the culture of the organization. As a result, individuals may model their behavior after these persons, for better or worse. The leader's influence ought never to be underestimated.

The third group of individuals refers to those with whom we have established relationships from other organizations. For example, one may have relationships with individuals from different provinces, states or countries. These relationships, though more distant than the former two categories, may nonetheless have a role to play in how we deal with ethical issues.

III. Issue-Specific Moderators—The Ethical Intensity of the Issue

The nature of the decision itself may have an impact upon the way in which we approach ethical dilemmas (e.g., Jones, 1991). Some issues simply may not be ethically contentious and require very little, if any, ethical consideration. On the other hand, some issues may be ethically loaded and the failure to recognize the moral intensity may result in dramatic outcomes for the individual and the organization. The moderators to be discussed in this section will help with the exploration of the ethical intensity of a dilemma. This will help us to decide the relative intellectual demands required of the decision-maker (the more ethically intense, the more ethically demanding).

1. Normative Consensus. The decision-maker's awareness of the general perception of the group or community regarding a particular issue will help in deciding its relative ethical intensity. For example, if a doctor is practicing in a strongly fundamentalist Christian community, the decision to open a clinic in which abortions could be conducted would be much more ethically intense than would a decision to offer polio vaccinations. The community's concern may (or should) heighten the level of the decision-maker's ethical reasoning regarding the particular issue.

This is not to say that the norms of the community are necessarily right or good and must be followed. The caveat here is that the community's opinion will determine only the relative support or conflict that the decision-maker will have when he or she acts. The group has been known to be terribly wrong, as Socrates and Galileo experienced first hand!

2. Physical and Psychological Distance. The distance, physical or psychological, which separates the individual from the dilemma can have an effect upon the decision-maker's perception of ethical intensity. If an issue has occurred in a distant location, the decision-maker may not be compelled to act to the same degree as she or he would if the issue occurred locally. For example, the HIV blood scandal that occurred in France in the 1990s may have relatively little influence upon the manner in which blood is handled in South Africa or in Belize, Central America.

Psychological distance refers to the extent to which the decision-maker is intimately involved with the issue or the circumstances surrounding it. When a doctor is required to operate, it is presumably more difficult to remain objective if the patient is related to the physician.

3. Magnitude of the Consequences. This moderator refers to the potential impact of the ethical issue upon the public or the individual. An issue that will result in very little negative or positive outcome is obviously less contentious and demanding than one that causes a great deal of harm or good. For example, the magnitude of consequence for a health administrator inadvertently securing incompetent student volunteers to distribute coffee and tea will have less negative impact upon the patients in the hospital than would the potential harm of hiring an incompetent surgeon. The former will create some social discomfort, while the latter may result in fatalities.

Simply, a full analysis of the impact is part of any decision-making strategy. Included in this type of analysis is consideration of the positive and negative outcomes of different possible ways in which to proceed. Central to this process is a sound ethical basis from which to weigh the outcomes in both directions.

4. Probability of Effect. This variable refers to the likelihood that a good or bad outcome of an action will actually occur. The greater the likelihood of an outcome taking place, the greater the moral intensity; the less likely, the less morally intensive. For example, the choice of a surgical procedure that has a moderate success rate for patients is less ethically intensive than the decision to attempt a more radical, yet theoretically superior, experimental procedure. In the former case, the probability of positive effect is rated as moderate; in the latter, the probability of positive or negative effect is empirically unknown.

5. Concentration of Effect. The extent to which good or harm is potentially distributed may influence a decision-maker's reasoning behavior. If the good or harm is distributed over a great number of individuals and everyone is affected minimally, it may be less contentious than if it affects one person severely. For example, suppose pharmaceutical Company A introduces a vitamin supplement that is safe, yet results in some minor intestinal discomfort for most users (it is effective but uncomfortable). Company B introduces a supplement that is more complex than Company A's vitamin, but may result in some liver dysfunction for 3% of long-term users (extremely effective yet potentially dangerous for a minority of individuals). The concentration of effect of Company A's product is less than that of Company B's product.

This variable has wide-ranging and diverse ramifications for all professional practices. Regardless of what aspect of public health we are engaged in, there is constant and great potential to influence so many by what we do. As a result, we cannot ignore or partition the fundamental role ethics plays in our decision-making behavior.

6. Immediacy. The time constraint placed upon the decision-maker may heighten or lessen the perceived intensity of an ethical dilemma. An issue that must be resolved immediately will undoubtedly hone the decision-maker's reasoning capacity to a greater degree than a resolution that can be delayed. For example, to remove an abusive health care worker from the public is far more ethically pressing than the decision to develop a policy of professional conduct. Both are necessary; the former requires immediate attention, while the latter does not.

7. Strategic or Tactical Decision. The final moderator of ethical intensity describes the difference between strategic and tactical decisions. Strategic decisions deal with long-term and more global issues of the hospital or organization's functioning. The decisions that concern the organizational culture are typically strategic. The decisions that focus upon the day-to-day operations of the hospital or organization are tactical. While both categories of decisions must be given attention, the implication of strategic decisions arguably transcends tactical ones and, therefore, must be given considerably more cognitive regard. For example, the decision to develop a mission statement for the hospital (i.e., strategic) demands greater attention and is ethically more laden than a decision to change the public access to the cafeteria.

IV. Organizational (Cultural) Moderators of Ethical Decision Making

Cultural moderators refer to the ideology, the explicit values, the observable behavior of members and the physical structures of an organization. Together, these moderators combine to form what many call "the way we do things around here." Culture, in this usage, does not necessarily refer to ethnic culture. However, as discussed previously, ethnicity may play a role in the manner in which organizational members perceive and act ethically.

1. Ideology. The ideology of an organization represents the philosophical basis for its culture. It consists of the implicit or unquestioned rationale for the existence of the organization. This may include the assumptions relating to the interaction with and relationship to the physical environment; the perceived nature and purpose of human activity; the nature of human relationships, both internal and external to the organization; and the perception of time, of reality and of truth. These assumptions define the basic premises upon which the organization evolves and, ultimately, revolves.

2. Values. Values are another essential feature of organizational culture. If ideology is the "blueprint" of organizational culture, we might consider values as the culture's conceptual "building blocks."

One definition of a value is that it is a concept of the desirable with a motivating force. This definition implies that a value is something abstract; that is, it is something that humans create, both for themselves and for their organizations. In addition, if a value is deemed desirable, this suggests that it is acceptable by most. Thus, when we speak of values, the desire of the group outweighs, usually, the desire of the individual. Finally, a value motivates us to do something.

A strongly held value will push us to behave in a particular manner. If, for example, an organizational value is client service, members may be motivated to behave in order to ensure that clients/patients feel welcome, comfortable, confident and safe within the jurisdiction of the health organization. Thus you can surmise that organizational values have a significant role to play in understanding what and why we do what we do.

We must also consider the extent to which a match exists between formal and informal organizational values. Formal values are those that are publicly and officially promoted by the organization. Informal values are those that are not officially pronounced, yet are integral to the daily functioning of the organization.

The extent to which there is a match between formal and informal value structures will determine the relative strength of the culture of the organization. Overall, if all individuals are operating from the same "blueprint," if they are using the same conceptual "building blocks," then the organization will, ideally, be more effective in accomplishing its goals. Should there not be a match, conflict may follow and the efficiency, effectiveness and perhaps the humanistic aspect of the organization may suffer.

The physical structures of the organization provide us with another aspect or frame of culture. The things around us show where we place value. Does a children's ward in a hospital have a display of patients' drawings? Does it have a display case for public donors or employees of the month? Is the hospital clean and safe? Are members provided with the equipment necessary to accomplish their task? These physical items are often tangible indicators of the ideology and values of the organization being put into action.

It has been argued that the fundamental role of leadership in organizational culture is its further development and maintenance. This responsibility is perhaps a new dimension to be considered by many. It may be common sense to others. Nonetheless, attending to the development of ethical culture and its maintenance through the "frames" of ideology, values and structures can result in effective, holistic, human and humane organizational functioning.

V. External Moderators of Ethical Decision Making

External moderators consist of those variables that are outside the confines of the organization. These moderators include technology, economics, politics and society. These moderators may influence, to a greater or lesser extent, the actual decision-making behavior of the individual. They have been placed at the periphery of the model (Figure 5.1) to suggest less intense influence than moderators more centrally situated. Despite this conceptual location, the impact of these moderators can be extremely powerful.

1. Technology. The impact that new innovations may have upon human behavior can be significant. The ability to genetically alter DNA strands, for example, creates many more ethical dilemmas than were present a decade ago. From this perspective, it is critical that our ethical awareness, our ability to recognize ethically contentious issues, keeps pace with the rapid development of technology. In other words, while we celebrate the achievement of research, we must also temper the application and implication of new discoveries with respect for humanity.

2. Economy. Economic moderators influence the availability or scarcity of resources available to health care. The relative scarcity of resources creates an environment of competition and rationalization. It is typically in such competitive situations that unethical practices may occur. In tough economic times, the number of hospital beds is reduced, elective surgery is limited, hospital stays are shortened and staff is overworked. The health administrator's challenge is to not only consider the "bottom line" of his or her budget, but also to consider the quality of care that is acceptable for the individual as patient.

3. Politics. The political realm deals with power. Power may manifest itself in terms of the influence that political parties attempt to garner from voters concerned about health care policy, as well as in legislation that controls the practices and parameters of health care professionals. Politics, like economics, deals in scarce resources, and those who are able to wield power are those that control the destiny of the health care system for good or bad, right or wrong. For example, recent legislation in the Canadian province of British Columbia has attempted to open the door for the provincial government to sue tobacco companies for the costs of treatment for those who are ill from smoking. Such legislation has tremendous implications, not only for the legal and health care system, but also for the notion of individual agency and decision-making responsibility.

4. Society. The norms which are held by society provide a framework for much of what we consider to be ethical. This is of considerable importance, as much of the population, according to cognitive structural psychologists, base their notion of ethical conduct upon the norms of significant others and/or society in general. Societal norms and values shape what policy is defended, critiqued and developed. It determines what is valued and what is valuable generally. Societal norms are fluid, and as such, the consensus among the public of what is ethically contentious is equally situational. An obvious illustration is the "pro-choice" movement that has risen in direct relation to the feminist movement. Though this issue continues to create a tremendous amount of debate, the fact that women consider having the choice to control their bodies is a massive change in perspective from the past.

VI. Interaction Effect

The moderators we have thus far discussed in the model have been presented as layers surrounding a core of the decision-making process. To clarify the relations among these layers we present the following four propositions:

Proposition 1. The arrangement of the layers implies that those moderators closest to the core have potentially greater influence upon the process of ethical decision making than do those more distally from the core. Despite this logic, we suggest that typically the process may be influenced to a greater extent by distal layers or moderators than proximal ones. For example, though an organizational culture may pressure an individual to behave in a particular manner, the influence of this person's church may hold more relative power of persuasion. The point made here is that, although there exists some logic to a rather linear arrangement of moderators, this logic may not always hold and the decision-maker must be prepared for the unexpected.

Proposition 2. The extent to which any moderator influences the ethical process will be mediated by individual moderators. For example, those reasoning from a conventional realm will be influenced to a much greater extent than those functioning from a post-conventional level. The deontologist will be affected to a greater degree by organizational policy than will the existentialist or the teleologist.

Proposition 3. The actual decisions, particularly those generated from the core, can influence each moderator surrounding it. An individual's decision might affect in a profound way the behavior of significant others, the organization's culture, and perhaps even the societal or political structure generally.

Proposition 4. Moderators can influence each other reciprocally. For example, organizational culture can influence the behavior of significant others as well as a variety of external moderators and, in turn, may be influenced by them. Thus there is influence being generated toward the core, between layers of the model and also from the core to external layers.

***

In this chapter we have identified five layers of moderators that may influence, to a greater or lesser extent, the decision-making process. Each layer represents a set of variables that should be considered in order for the individual to fully understand the complexity, breadth and significance of decision-making behavior. While the significance of each layer will vary according to the nuances of any particular case presented in Chapter 9 or actual issue faced outside the classroom, the model we have presented provides the reader with a framework from which comprehensive ethical decisions can be made. In the next chapter, a process of ethical decision making is introduced which expands upon the core of the model presented here.

6

The Process of Ethical Decision Making

In the previous chapter, we discussed many variables or moderators that may, to a greater or lesser extent, influence the manner in which we make ethical or unethical decisions. In this chapter we look at a process of ethical decision making that will provide the reader with a more comprehensive analysis and plan of ethics-in-action.

The use of any particular decision-making model will not always guarantee the best decision. The result depends on the decision-maker's ethical beliefs, cognitive abilities, intentions and creativity. Having said this, we present the following as a framework for the analysis and development of a logical, consistent and comprehensive ethical decision.

The process consists of seven stages (Figure 6.1). Within each stage, the reader is urged to consider the analysis from three separate ethical perspectives—teleology (good)) deontology (right) and existentialism (authentic). By using this unique three-way ethical analysis, the reader assesses a particular dilemma in a more comprehensive way than by using only one theory or process or employing no conscious ethical stance at all (as is the typical manner in which most case studies are analyzed). The result is a better and conscious ethical decision that is good, right and authentic.

The Seven Stages

1. Recognition of the Ethical Dilemma or Cause. The first stage of the process is the actual acknowledgment that there is, in fact, a dilemma, and that it is ethically laden. If an individual perceives that an issue is in need of resolution, yet does not see its ethical nature, an attempt to solve the problem will go on without the insight of a conscious and comprehensive investigation of ethics. The problem is then solved with the decision-maker using an unconscious ethical bias. For example, as explained earlier, one may use, without examination, a teleological perspective to solve the dilemma. As a result, all the pitfalls of using this theory exclusively will befall the decision-maker (i.e., ends justifying means) and a relatively narrow resolution will be the outcome.

Figure 6.1: A Process for Ethical Decision Making

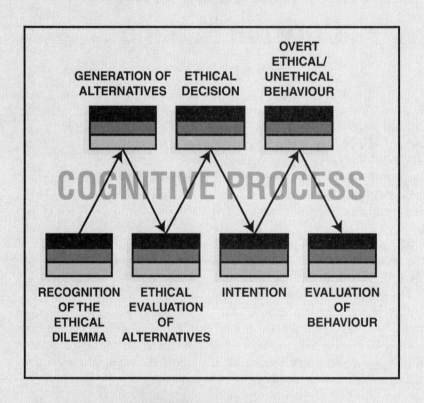

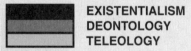

Therefore, the initial stage in the process is an all-important one in order for the remaining six stages to contribute meaning to a good, right and authentic ethical decision.

The *teleological recognition* will focus upon the degree to which the best ends are achieved for the group (utilitarianism) or the individual (hedonism). The decision-maker must assess the extent to which the dilemma presents barriers to the accomplishment of group or individual goals. The following questions may help the decision-maker in determining the teleological basis of the dilemma.

1. Does the dilemma prevent ends from being achieved for the individual?

2. Does the dilemma prevent ends from being achieved for the group?

These very simple questions provide the basis of teleological recognition.

The *deontological recognition* will focus upon the rules that have or have not been followed and the duty, implicit or explicit, which has or has not been assumed. The decision-maker may wish to ask the following questions to decide whether rules or duty are at issue.

1. (a) Has a rule, a policy, a procedure or a code of ethics been broken?
   (b) Is it a bad rule, policy, procedure or a code that ought to be broken?

2. (a) Has a law been broken?
   (b) Is it a bad law that ought to be changed?

3. What was the implicit and explicit duty of individuals in the case?

4. Was this sense of duty followed?

The issues these questions raise will provide the decision-maker with some needed information to determine the deontological aspect of dilemma recognition.

The *existential recognition* will focus upon the extent to which the dilemma has created a situation in which some aspect of the individual's authenticity is being restricted or denied. The decision-maker may wish to ask the following questions to determine whether authenticity is at issue.

1. Is there a restriction upon the individual's freedom to choose?

2. Is there a restriction upon the individual's freedom to take responsibility for action?

3. Is there an attempt in general to control an individual's or a group's behavior?

4. Is there an attempt to deny an individual's free will?

If any one of these questions can be answered positively then the dilemma has been recognized as having an existential feature. Eventually the decision-maker must address this feature through the choice of resolutions.

Through the perspectives of each ethical theory, the reader can discover a wide range of possible problems. Once each of these perspectives has been examined, the reader must then decide what, in fact, is the actual problem or cause. It may be that the problem is complex; a mosaic of subproblems. However, the reader must detect which problem is the cause of the others. So often students analyzing cases make the error of identifying the first problem they discover and assume that it is, in fact, the issue to be addressed. Without careful consideration, students may choose a symptom of the primary cause rather than addressing the actual nub of the ethical dilemma. As a result the analysis proceeds, the symptom is resolved, yet the primary issue remains unresolved. Therefore it is important that the reader is convinced that the problem identified is in fact the cause of all symptoms and not a symptom of a greater cause. (See D.C. Malloy and D.L. Lang, 1993. "An Aristotelian approach to case study analysis," *Journal of Business Ethics* 12:511-16.)

2. Generation of Alternatives. The second stage of the process is the generation of alternative solutions based upon the tenets of each of the three ethical perspectives. The rationale, to reiterate, is to be ethically comprehensive at each stage of the process to provide good, right and authentic solutions. The decision-maker must, therefore, develop plausible alternatives for the resolution of the dilemma from teleological, deontological and existential positions.

The teleological position will be geared toward achieving group or individual ends. The deontological position will focus upon rules, policies and duty. The existential position will contribute alternatives that involve free will and choice, responsibility and authenticity. The intent of this stage is not necessarily to be locked into a particular school of thought. It is quite probable and desirable that alternatives be composed of two or all three ethical positions, that is, alternatives that can resolve the dilemma in a good, right and authentic manner. The reader may wish to generate alternatives from each position separately before attempting an amalgamation of two or more positions. Being locked into one ethical orientation may result in a constricted, rather than a comprehensive and rich, ethical analysis. This phase requires a great deal of effort and creativity from the reader, for it is from this stage that the eventual resolution to the dilemma arises. As Hodgkinson (1983) states, sometimes "he who does not hesitate [and reflect/examine] is lost" (p.104).

3. Evaluation of Alternatives. The third stage of the process is the evaluation of alternatives. Each alternative is assessed, based upon the criteria of the three ethical theories. The decision-maker has to decide to what extent each alternative is good, right and authentic. That is, does it accomplish the best end; does it follow or create a rule, a policy, a procedure or a law? Does it allow the individual to be free to choose and to be responsible for all action? The alternative that best satisfies these criteria in the most comprehensive manner is presumably the ideal alternative to select.

4. Selection of the Ideal Solution. To restate, the ideal solution is the option that is the most comprehensively good, right and authentic. The identification of the ideal or comprehensive alternative does not necessarily result in the use of the ideal solution. In any organizational setting, there will be many pressures and surprises that come up unexpectedly; the world of human interaction is often in a state of subtle or blatant chaos. These moderators, which upset the ideal or theoretical process, may influence the intent of the decision-maker to start the ideal solution.

5. Intention. One's intent, according to Aristotle and Kant, is perhaps the strongest determinant of ethical action. If your intention is to carry out an ideal resolution, then presumably and conceptually you will. Unless unforeseen circumstances that are beyond your control prevent you from doing so, the ideal decision will become the actual decision. If, however, your intention is not to carry out the ideal solution because of a variety of moderators (e.g., peer pressure, moral intensity, organizational climate and culture or societal pressure), then the actual decision will differ from the ideal. For example, suppose that you have worked through the decision process and determine that the good, right and authentic decision for a hospital fundraising program is to prohibit funding from tobacco or alcohol sponsors. However, by doing so you will undoubtedly be the focus of the wrath of various powerful board members who demand a successful fundraising campaign whatever the ethics involved. Not only could you lose your job, but the hospital will suffer, and some valuable traditional sources of revenue will be lost. As you have no immediate job opportunities at hand and your young family is dependent upon you, you choose not to carry out the ideal solution and opt instead for a weaker or watered-down resolution.

6. The Actual Decision. The actual decision is, one would hope, the most comprehensively ethical decision. That is, it is good, right and authentic. The actual decision is a function or product of the individual's discovery of the ideal decision, the moderating variables that will allow its implementation and the individual intent to carry through with the ethical choice. The decision may or may not satisfy all criteria. However, this process has provided the decision-maker with the logic to consider a variety of perspectives that have ultimately resulted in a comprehensive and informed or conscious resolution.

Figure 6.2: Summary of Case Study Analysis

THE MODERATORS

1. **Individual**: ethical orientation; level of moral development; demographic variables.

2. **Issue-Specific**: normative consensus; physical and psychological distance; magnitude of consequence; probability of effect; concentration of effect; immediacy, strategic/tactical orientation.

3. **Significant Other:** personal; interorganizational; extraorganizational.

4. **Situational:** organizational ideology; organizational culture and climate.

5. **External:** political; economic; technical; societal.

THE PROCESS

6. Identify the problem from each perspective.

7. Develop alternatives from each perspective.

8. Evaluate each alternative from each perspective.

9. Select the ideal solution.

10. Determine intention to act upon the ideal solution.

11. Actual decision.

12. Evaluation of the actual decision from each perspective.

7. Evaluation of the Actual Decision. As we have stated throughout this text, the decision-maker should seek to make good, right and authentic decisions. At this point in the analysis, you must decide the extent to which the actual decision has met the comprehensive ethical criteria. Does it accomplish desired ends? Does it follow existing rules or have new ones been made? Does it allow for individual free will and the accompanying responsibility? If the actual decision does not meet each of the three criteria, can the decision-maker justify this less than comprehensive resolution? For example, perhaps a decision was made that was right and authentic, yet was not good. In other words, the decision followed the rules, was true to the decision-maker's heart, but did not accomplish the intended goals. Can such a decision be defended?

To conclude, we urge the reader to seek comprehensive ethical solutions that are good, right and authentic. We also caution that such a comprehensive resolution may be difficult, if possible or desirable, to achieve. Figure 6.2 provides a summary of the moderators and process of this second model. While we believe that each of these stages of ethical analysis are extremely important, the reader is well advised to make use of those moderators which are pertinent to the dilemma or case study at hand. An example of the application of this second model is provided in Chapter 9.

7

Biomedical Ethical Principles

To enable you to engage in moral discourse on a higher level than ordinary dialogue, a number of introductory concepts in ethics (moral philosophy) have been discussed. Basic definitions have been presented to clarify concepts and establish common understandings for terms generally known but used in diverse ways. The importance of selecting and enunciating an ethical maxim, to be used as the agreed-upon yardstick or standard against which behavior is to be measured, has been emphasized. Three ethical theories—consequential, non-consequential and existentialism—have been outlined to elucidate their applicability to the human condition. Each one can serve as a source from which an ethical maxim can be derived. Two models—one, more basic, and the other, more encompassing, since it includes psychological and social modifiers—have been presented to guide step-by-step moral reasoning. Using either or both models will enable the health care professional to render moral judgment as the end result of a thoughtful, analytical, critical and comprehensive process.

The case for the need for health care professionals to render moral judgment on an almost continuous basis has been made and hence need not be repeated here. However, in order to improve the newly acquired moral reasoning skills, practice is needed. As each case study is addressed, ample opportunity to practice will be provided. Before actually dealing with the case studies, two additional factors need to be considered: (1) the five basic medical principles, and (2) models of medical practice. These medical principles, ethical in nature, serve to guide practice, and each of the models of medical practice embodies a somewhat different set of values. The set of medical principles and the models of medical practice must be taken into account, since elements of both will be influential factors in the moral judgment rendered.

Five Biomedical Ethical Principles

Since its inception some 2,500 years ago, the Hippocratic oath has incorporated ethical principles which serve to guide the practice of medicine and, by logical extension, apply to the allied health care fields. Three principles em-

bedded in the Hippocratic oath are readily discernible. These are nonmaleficence, beneficence and confidentiality, and they continue to serve as ethical
guides. In contemporary times, in part under the influence of the nascent
patient's rights movement, respect for individual autonomy has been added to
the list along with the notion of justice. Each will be outlined briefly.

Nonmaleficence

Nonmaleficence may be regarded as the most basic principle. It can be
summed up in the phrase "first do no harm." There is a professional obligation
not to inflict harm and, whenever possible, to prevent harm. Physicians are
proscribed from doing anything intentionally that will harm the patient. As
important as this advice sounds, the dictum is not absolute. There are occasions when "inflicting harm" cannot be avoided for the greater good of the
patient. A gangrenous leg must be amputated in order to save the life of the
patient. All surgery, from a very superficial perspective, can be labeled as
harm, but when the greater good of the patient is considered, it is apparent that
the harm done is actually a good, a procedure which is designed to avert
greater harm in the future.

Not all cases are as clear-cut as amputating a gangrenous limb. Far more
problematic is the case of a baby born with spina bifida. What does nonmaleficence mean in such a situation, particularly in the context of the values
expressed in the phrases "sanctity of life" and "quality of life"? Will less harm
be done if there is no medical intervention, thus allowing nature to take its
course? This path averts repeated major surgery in the future, with its attendant pain and anguish for all concerned. In contrast, a physician committed to
the notion of sanctity of life would support doing everything to prolong life.

At least two additional issues emerge from the questions posed. What is
meant by ordinary and extraordinary care within the context of nonmaleficence? And secondly, as will be outlined in the next section, each of the
diverse models of medical practice contains varying values which would tend
to interpret nonmaleficence in different ways.

Beneficence

Beneficence is the extension of nonmaleficence; it is an affirmative duty
requiring the physician to take action for the good of the patient. The physician is duty-bound to relieve pain and suffering, to restore health and preserve
life. In its broadest sense, beneficence means there is a duty to do good.

In contemporary times, beneficence may also be interpreted to mean
spending time counseling patients, particularly urging a change in lifestyle to
include proper diet and exercise (Physical Activity and Health: A report of the
Surgeon General, 1996). Counselling patients in this manner falls under the
heading of preventive medicine. The issue of remuneration arises here, since

neither governments nor private insurance companies recognize this type of "treatment" in their fee schedules. But, as will be discussed shortly (under the heading of Justice), changes in lifestyle will reduce demands on the health care delivery system, thus making more resources available to the seriously ill.

Knowing one's own limitations regarding the ability to diagnose and treat, and knowing when to refer a patient to a specialist, may also fall under the heading of beneficence.

Confidentiality

Confidentiality restricts what use can be made of the information obtained from the patient by the physician. As the patient imparts information to the physician, there is some "invasion of privacy." This knowledge is privileged information, to be guarded carefully; it must not become public except under extraordinary circumstances. Information about the patient must not be divulged to others where there is an understanding, either explicit or implicit, not to reveal it. Permission of the patient is required before the physician can release the information.

Absolute confidentiality is problematic when consideration is given to the need to balance the interests of the patient with the protection of society. To gain and maintain the trust of patients, physicians must assure them that complete confidentiality will be maintained. There are times when patients, under treatment, have vowed to either assault or murder someone. When that occurs, the physician is faced with a confounding moral dilemma. Alerting the police is a breach of confidentiality, a breach of trust, but remaining silent imperils the safety of others, since harm will be inflicted on them. The principles of nonmaleficence and beneficence are implicated here. Unfortunately there are a number of actual cases reported in the literature (the one cited most often is Tarasoff, California Supreme Court, 1976) where the physician's adherence to confidentiality resulted in the death of others and subsequently greater harm to the patient.

Maintaining strict confidentiality may conflict with the law. In certain political jurisdictions, physicians are bound, legally, to report cases where they suspect injuries to children have resulted from abusive behavior by adults. Physicians cannot violate the law with impunity; such cases must be reported even if it means confidentiality has been breached.

Respect for Individual Autonomy

In the time of Hippocrates, and for many centuries thereafter, a strong paternalistic attitude pervaded the practice of medicine; the physician knew what was best for the patient and administered treatment without even bothering to obtain approval first. Today the situation is much different. Autonomy may be conceptualized as respect for the individuality and personhood of the patient. It can also be described as a form of personal liberty where patients determine their own course of action.

Rooted in Kant's categorical imperative, the notion of respect for autonomy imposes a moral obligation on the physician to treat others as "ends in themselves" and never as merely means. Patients are acknowledged as adults (except, obviously, when the patient is a child), capable of making decisions about what affects them. It is the patient who has the final say regarding treatment, even when those decisions are contrary to what is recommended by the physician. Where there is a disagreement, the patient, if competent and sound of mind, is the final authority. Respect for autonomy can clash with the notions of nonmaleficence and beneficence.

Patients need to be consulted (except in obvious situations, such as unconsciousness, where consultation cannot take place) and their consent obtained prior to treatment. Obtaining consent presumes that the patient is competent to make decisions based on an explanation given that is comprehensible. Information needs to be conveyed in plain language rather than in technical terms; the likelihood of treatment succeeding needs to be discussed; the potential side-effects need to be mentioned; the anticipated consequences need to be identified; and the costs involved, both monetary and emotional, need to be communicated. This information should be presented in a way that enables the patient to make a decision that is authentic for himself or herself.

Care must be taken not to overwhelm the patient with too many facts and questions. A clinician ought to offer options and assist the patient in finding the right course for the management of his or her condition. At times, the patient will cede decision-making authority to someone else, for example a spouse or relative. That choice needs to be respected by the clinician. Ethically, the physician is bound to accept the decision made by the patient, even if the choice is refusal of treatment.

Justice

Justice, when implemented as a principle, means that medical resources will be allocated fairly. Distributive justice, rather than corrective or retributive, is the applicable notion. This understanding takes into account greater needs, which are then given immediate attention. When all factors are considered, equals should be treated equally and unequals unequally. Due to cutbacks in funds allocated to health care, some rather severe, both by governments (where applicable) and by private insurers (where applicable), the concept of justice as fair and equitable allocation of medical resources will be tested much more now (and in the future, if the present trend continues) than in the past.

These five ethical principles serve to guide medical practice and together provide a specific context within which the case studies in the next chapter are analyzed and assessed.

Models of Medical Practice

Scholars have examined the practice of medicine and, as they discerned certain patterns, a number of models were delineated. Each model described reflects a different conception of medicine and is undergirded by a different complex of values. Consideration given to these models, that is, to the actual practice of medicine, provides an additional context within which to discuss the case studies.

Three models of medical practice are identified and described briefly by Sass (1990): the Hippocratic model, the contractual model and the partner model. The Hippocratic model is the traditional one, where the physician is morally bound to help fellow human beings who are ill or in pain and need medical attention. A somewhat different situation prevails in the second (contractual) model: The physician is the provider and the patient is the recipient of specialized service. Within this model, the patient has full autonomy and the physician-patient relationship is basically the same as in other provider-client relationships. In the third (partner) model, the physician is seen more as the patient's consultant and together, as partners, they manage the health of the patient. There are subtle differences in the role of the physician and, consequently, in the role of the patient, particularly regarding the amount of responsibility assumed by each. As more responsibility is assumed by the patient, the role of the physician changes.

Three somewhat different models are outlined by Francoeur (1983): the engineering model, the paternalistic model and the social contract model. In the engineering model, the physician assumes the role of the detached scientist who is uninvolved emotionally with the patient and the process. As scientists, they are removed from all questions of values and deal only with the facts. The facts are presented to the patient, who then assumes full responsibility for making all decisions. Once the decisions are made, the physician executes the wishes of the patient, whatever they may be, even if such action is contrary to the physician's own set of values (e.g., performing an abortion).

The paternalistic model is well known: The physician, acting in the role of wise parent, makes decisions which are deemed to be in the best interest of the patient. Consulting the patient and obtaining input is done only when the physician thinks it is in the best interest of the patient. This model is somewhat similar to the Hippocratic model as outlined by Sass.

The social contract model takes its name from the implicit contract which comes into existence whenever one human being needs help from another or seeks advice, and the other, more knowledgeable, person agrees to help. As

Figure 7.1: English's Models of Medical Practice

1. **Engineering Model.** This model was identified by Francoeur and its features were discussed in the text.

2. **Priestly Model.** This is similar to the paternalistic model mentioned above but extends beyond medicine to offering advice to the patient on how to behave in all aspects of life. In this model, the patient assumes a dependency role.

3. **Collegial Model.** This is similar to the partnership model; physician and patient are colleagues in the mutual pursuit of healing. Contributions from both parties are valued.

4. **Contractual Model.** This is similar to the model of the same name described by Sass. As English (1994) notes, "limited obligations and benefits are negotiated and shared; basic norms of freedom, dignity, truth telling, promise keeping, and justice are essential" (p.13). Agreement is reached between physician and patient on how to proceed while maintaining autonomy and respecting the personhood of all parties involved.

5. **Authoritarian Model.** This model extends beyond the paternalistic, since the physician is reluctant to share much with the patient. Within this model, the physician shoulders almost all the responsibility and often issues directives regarding patient care and behavior. It is the responsibility of the patient to carry out the instructions given by the physician.

6. **Warrior Model.** Within this model, the physician wages war against the enemy, disease and trauma, with the patient's body as the battleground. A serious concern is expressed by English (1994) about patient passivity in this model.

7. **Managerial Model.** This is similar to the contractual relationship, but here there is clear acknowledgment that, should the need arise, other physicians, or other health care professionals with more specialized knowledge, will become involved.

8. **Entrepreneurial Model.** Within this model, one of the goals of the physician is to maximize income. Without doubting that competent, socially acceptable care can be provided, a certain tension must exist if income maximization is the main goal. An inherent conflict of interest is present whenever the interest of the patient is not placed ahead of billing considerations.

Francoeur describes this model, which relies on mutual obligations and rights, it appears to be similar to the partner model as outlined by Sass.

The most encompassing treatment is provided by English (1994) who identifies and briefly outlines eight models. He also points out that these models may reflect certain personality types and hence are chosen by certain physicians (see Figure 7.1).

***

In conclusion, various models of medical practice exist. Those outlined above were derived from observing how physicians conduct themselves. Each model has advantages and drawbacks for both the practitioner and patient. Personality factors are involved as well; some physicians are more comfortable practicing in one way than in another. How one practices is a reflection of a personal set of values and that, in turn, is a factor which will emerge during the moral discourse undertaken as each case in Chapter 9 is analyzed and assessed.

8

Putting Theory into Action

In this chapter we will apply our models to an actual case study (see Figure 8.1). The case, which is based on an actual event, involves ethical issues with respect to the decision to operate on a patient. As the steps and elements of Model I are applied, the exercise will serve as a template for the conduct of moral discourse. A trial-run with Model II follows immediately after.

A Trial Run with Model I

The behavior of both individuals, Dr. M.J., the resident, and Dr. D.K., the surgeon, merit scrutiny.

Step One—Obtain and Clarify All the Pertinent Facts

As the first step in the process, a request is made to determine if anyone present, perchance, can provide more information about the case.

Since the case is straightforward, clarification is not needed.

Step Two—Identify and Enunciate the Ethical Maxim(s)

Three ethical bases (or theories)—consequentialism, non-consequentialism and existentialism—have been identified as the sources from which ethical maxims can be derived. In addition, the five ethical principles (Chapter 7) which guide the practice of medicine can also serve in this capacity. From that source—nonmaleficence and beneficence—one ethical maxim can be identified immediately: what is best for the patient?

From a deontological source, it appears that there are no written rules regarding how an attending surgeon is to treat a resident. There is a general policy which, most often, is stated in broad terms: provision of the best possible education for residents. Since such statements, where they actually exist, are amenable to many interpretations, it is difficult to see how a specifically worded ethical maxim can be derived from that policy.

From an existential perspective, an ethical maxim can be derived which applies to both the resident and the surgeon: Did each behave in an authentic fashion? Were they true to their own nature?

Figure 8.1: TRIAL-RUN CASE—The Need to Operate

Dr. M.J., a resident mid-way through her program, arrives at a new hospital and is assigned to Dr. D.K., a surgeon with a generally fine reputation. In the first case she deals with, Dr. D.K., after an examination, advises the patient of the urgent need to operate. Very little additional information is presented to the patient other than that Dr. M.J. would perform her own examination. At the end of her examination, Dr. M.J. is convinced that the procedure prescribed by Dr. D.K. is not absolutely necessary as described by the attending surgeon; in her opinion the illness can be, indeed ought to be, treated with medication. She expresses her views to Dr. D.K., who is adamant that his diagnosis and decision is the proper one. He points to the potential side-effects of the suggested medications and the continued discomfort of the patient. Immediate surgery would not only cure the illness, but it would also put an end to the discomfort.

During the discussion, Dr. D.K. asserts that he will not have his professional judgment questioned by a student. If she is really there to learn, she should listen attentively to him, thus benefiting from his vast experience and fund of knowledge.

Despite his tirade, Dr. M.J. is still convinced that surgery is not the best treatment in this case and begins to wonder about how she will fare in this rotation.

As she ponders the case, another issue, remuneration, floats to consciousness. Payment for performing surgery is much higher than treatment with medication, even with its attendant ongoing monitoring which has the additional drawback of being more time-consuming.

(1) She wonders if she should report the matter to the chief of surgery at the hospital. That step would necessitate going over the head of the surgeon, who, at the end of the rotation, will write her evaluation, a report which will have considerable impact on her career.

(2) She also wonders if she should report the matter to the Director of Graduate Medical Education at the university. That move would have other repercussions which would, once again, have potential adverse effects on her career.

After pondering the situation carefully, Dr. M.J. decides not to inform anyone and opts to heed the surgeon's directive: she will listen, observe and do as instructed.

To extend the exercise in order to invoke the use of the second model, a different scenario will be sketched. Dr. M.J. has ongoing contact with the patient. On the day prior to surgery, the patient asks Dr. M.J. for more information about the procedure. As the discussion evolves, the patient asks if there is an alternative to surgery available. Dr. Jones then must decide her course of action. She can state that she concurs with the opinion of Dr. D.K., leaving the impression that there is none. In the second scenario, she opines that the illness could be treated with medication instead of surgery.

Is surgery the best treatment for the patient? From a non-consequential perspective, no rule would seem to be broken if surgery were performed. However, two basic medical principles, nonmaleficence and beneficence, may be violated if a non-surgical procedure might be as effective as a treatment regimen. More medical details, which we do not have, are needed here in order to come to a proper conclusion.

Attempting to compare the two regimens leads us into the realm of conse-quentialism and the need to assess the amount of goodness and badness for the patient resulting from each procedure. Surgery is costly and painful and has some risks associated with it, but when it works, and once the patient recovers, normal life is resumed. Taking medication has some ongoing finan-cial costs as well as the potential for continuing discomfort. Assessing the total amount of goodness and badness resulting from each treatment regimen is a difficult challenge.

Another factor merits consideration from a consequentialist perspective: the remuneration received by the surgeon. More income earned is obviously preferable than less income earned. Should the financial benefits derived by the surgeon be factored into the total calculus of goodness and badness?

Did Dr. D.K. behave in an authentic manner by insisting surgery was the only treatment to consider? Did he behave properly toward the resident?

Did Dr. M.J. behave in an authentic manner by bringing her concerns regarding the treatment selected to Dr. D.K.?

Did she act in an authentic manner when she decided not to report the case to the Chief of Surgery or to the Director of Graduate Medical Education?

Step Three—Time

Attention is focused on (1) the time before the incident, (2) the time of the incident, and (3) the time after the incident. Questions about motivation and intention are posed.

Since we have no information about Dr. D.K.'s previous behavior, attention is directed to the time of the incident. What motivated him to recommend immediate surgery? Was remuneration a factor influencing the diagnosis? Was it his intention to provide the best medical care for the patient or was it maximizing income?

In the time following the incident, what motivated Dr. D.K. to treat his resident in an authoritarian way? What impact will this behavior have on the resident during the remainder of her time in that rotation? Will her learning be enhanced in such a relationship?

Step Four—Identify and Discuss Any Extenuating Circumstances

Given Dr. M.J.'s position as a student, dependent upon a good evaluation from Dr. D.K. to allow her to advance her career, was she justified in remaining silent?

Is this factor an extenuating circumstance?

Step Five—Render Judgment

Our goal in this exercise is to provide an example of how the steps in the model can be employed to examine all aspects of a case. This aim has now been achieved. In keeping with the views expressed at the beginning of the text, we refrain from rendering moral judgment for to do so would deprive the reader of the opportunity to come to an independent decision.

To extend the exercise (and complete the discussion), what judgment would you render if Dr. M.J. tells the patient she concurs with the opinion of Dr. D.K. that surgery is really required? What rationale would you use to support your stand?

What judgment would you render if Dr. M.J. advises the patient that an alternative non-surgical treatment is available? What rationale would you use to support your stand?

A Trial Run with Model II

In this section, we have provided a brief overview of how this case might be approached and what questions might be asked using the second model (see Figures 5.1 and 6.2 in previous chapters).

The Moderators

1. Individual Moderators. Though this case does not provide a great deal of information regarding the individual character of those involved, are there any interpretations or speculations you can make that would identify an ethical orientation of a level of moral development of Dr. M.J. or Dr. D.K. or the uninformed patient? Does the gender, age, informed knowledge or experience have a role to play?

2. Issue-Specific Moderators. This moderator can be expanded upon in detail by the student. Is there normative consensus for or against unnecessary surgery? By whom? Does the physical or psychological distance between Dr. M.J., Dr. D.K., and the patient have an effect? What possible positive or negative outcomes will result if the surgery is performed or not performed? Is the patient's well being an immediate concern? Is Dr. M.J.'s success on this particular rotation fundamental to her career?

3. Significant Other Moderator. Here there is much to discuss. The power relationship between the young female resident and the older male doctor may have tremendous impact upon the manner in which this dilemma can be resolved (and how it may be prevented from happening in the future). Are there other individuals that Dr. M.J. can access without fear of negative career implications? What external sources of advice, guidance or leadership can she seek?

4. Situational Moderators. Though there is little information provided with respect to organizational practices, what speculation can you offer about the formal or informal culture of the hospital, or the doctor-student environment? What policy is there that may cover an incident such as this? What are your thoughts about codes of ethics or whistle-blowing programs? Are they realistic? If not, how could they be?

5. External Moderators. What societal values may influence the current behavior and the subsequent resolution of the dilemma? What technical moderators are at play (i.e., surgical, medical)? Is there an economic motivation for the doctor? For the student? For the hospital? For society-at-large?

The Process

6. Identify the problem from each perspective. Would the consequentialist consider the dilemma as being an inefficient use of hospital resources and taxpayers money? Would the non-consequentialist consider it a problem where the patient is viewed as a means and not as an end? Would the existentialist be concerned with the lack of freedom (i.e., informed consent) provided to the patient?

7. Develop alternatives from each perspective. How would the consequentialist resolve the dilemma? The non-consequentialist? The existentialist? For example, Dr. M.J. could state that she concurs with the opinion of Dr. D.K. (i.e., abides by her non-consequentialist duty to follow orders of the superior or follows her hedonistic and preconventional impulse to save her career), leaving the impression that there is no other course of action than to operate; or she could admit that the illness is treatable with medication instead of surgery (perhaps a non-consequentialist, consequentialist, and/or existential perspective). Are there other alternatives that could be argued?

8. Evaluate each alternative from consequentialist, non-consequentialist and existential perspectives. Each alternative is screened through the ethical theories to identify strengths and weaknesses in order to allow for a reasoned choice in the next stage. How would you judge Dr. M.J.'s decision to say nothing? Existentially inauthentic? Non-consequentially weak or wrong? Consequentially bad (from the utilitarian view) or good (the hedonistic view)?

9. Select the ideal solution. This ideal solution is presumably a combination of the best of the good, the right and the authentic alternatives (i.e., it is a synthesis of the best consequentialist, non-consequentialist and existential alternatives).

10. Determine intention to act upon the ideal solution. As this particular case does not provide us with information regarding intention, it is difficult to comment but possible to speculate. It should be noted that this stage in the process is an essential one to consider when making actual ethical decisions outside the realm of the case study.

11. Actual decision. At this point the actual decision is determined, which may or may not be similar to Stage 10. In the second scenario provided in this case, we are free to speculate on what her eventual choice would be.

12. Evaluation of actual decision from consequentialist, non-consequentialist and existential perspectives. At this final stage of the process, the reader must determine whether or not the good, right and authentic has been achieved and then determine the rationale for its implementation. Was Dr. M.J.'s choice good? Right? Authentic? What are your thoughts regarding her options and her eventual decision?

***

In this chapter we have provided brief overviews of how a case could be approached using Model I and Model II. We would advise that those who are relatively unfamiliar with the realm of moral discourse should commence by using Model I as the basis for analysis. Once the reader becomes more familiar and perhaps more comfortable with ethics generally, then it is time to explore the cases to follow using the comprehensive Model II.

9

Case Studies

Introduction

A wide array of ethical issues are raised in the cases presented in this chapter. Each is an actual case. Whenever possible we have indicated the source of the report, but that could not be done in all instances. Certain situations are never reported by the mass media nor do they appear in the professional literature, yet these events have occurred and countless others, similar in nature, will occur in the future. As each case is considered, one or more of the five ethical principles which guide the practice of medicine (Chapter 7) is invoked. During the moral discourse, consideration needs to be given as to how, and why, they are implicated.

As the moral discourse evolves, it is expected that every participant will contribute to the discussion. Often the comments made will reflect that particular individual's set of values. At times what is uttered may come as a revelation to the speaker (as well as to the other members of the discussion group) because he or she had not been called upon previously to make pronouncements on such challenging and difficult issues. Yet these cases are representative of what awaits each member of the group in his or her future professional practice. Some of these dilemmas may have already been encountered during clerkship or residency or similar situations may be encountered the day following the discussion.

Discussion of the following cases will enable the participants to learn more about their own set of values; in part, the ethical analysis of each case is also an exercise in values clarification. As moral discourse evolves, most often general ethics, biomedical ethics, medical etiquette, personal beliefs, professional views and even economic forces intersect. At times the discussion may serve as the impetus for a reconsideration of one's own values and attitudes.

CASE 9.1
The Right to Live Longer

A decision made based on the principle of patient autonomy can place the physician in an awkward ethical position, one where traditional medical lore conflicts with the desires of the patient's family. This particular case serves as an example of one aspect of the physician-patient relationship and the concern for the broader good. A number of the biomedical principles are implicated here.

A hospital in a mid-western state resorted to court action to obtain permission to discontinue using a respirator on a patient. The patient, an 87-year-old comatose woman in a Persistent Vegetative State (PVS) secondary to a cardiac arrest and severe anoxic encephalopathy, had been on a respirator for more than a year. Her physicians all agreed that the continued use of a respirator was medically inappropriate and "non-beneficial." When the husband of the patient and her children were apprised of the physicians' decision, they refused to assent. They demanded that the use of a respirator be continued, because they believed in miracles and hoped that one would be forthcoming which would restore the patient's health. Care for the patient had cost the taxpayers and society more than $700,000 by the time the hospital filed court papers.

Questions to consider for discussion

1. What ethical basis is there for the patient's physicians to even consider a decision to remove the respirator?

2. From an ethical perspective, were the physicians right in concluding that the patient should be removed from the respirator?

3. What ethical basis is there for the patient's family insisting that the use of the respirator be continued, despite the enormous costs involved, while waiting for a miracle?

4. What justification can there be for spending $700,000 on one patient? What are the ethical implications for the rest of the community when so many resources are allocated to one patient?

5. What ethical basis is there for the hospital administrators' decision to take the case to court?

References

Angell, M. 1991. The case of Helga Wangle: A new kind of "right to die" case. *New England Journal Medicine* 325:511-512.

Brett, A.S., and L.B. McCullough. 1986. When patients request specific interventions: Defining the limits of the physician's obligation. *New England Journal Medicine* 315:1347-1351.

Clement, C.D., and R.C. Sider. 1993. Medical ethics' assault upon medical values. *Journal of the American Medical Association* 250:2011-2015.

Fischer, D.S. 1992. Observations on ethical problems and terminal care. *The Yale Journal of Biology and Medicine* 65:105-120.

Miles, S.H. 1990. Why a hospital seeks to discontinue care against family wishes. *Law, Medicine, Health Care* 18:424-425.

_____. 1991. Informed demand for "non-beneficial" medical treatment. *New England Journal Medicine* 325:512-515.

CASE 9.2

Who, Really, Has the Final Say?

Our current thinking regarding the central position of patient autonomy in medicine can be traced to the writings of Immanuel Kant and John Stuart Mill, along with many other philosophers of the Enlightenment era. This view sees the patient's right to determine his or her treatment as fundamental. A patient's refusal to undergo treatment often conflicts with the basic values of medicine, which strives to eliminate illness so that good health is restored. One important factor at play is the competence of the patient to make an informed decision. Who decides, and the basis used in making that decision, are factors which need to be taken into account in rendering moral judgment in this case.

A woman in her early fifties had a heart attack and, within four days, showed signs of acute mitral regurgitation. When cardiac catheterization was proposed, she initially refused but upon reconsideration agreed to the procedure. Based on the information garnered, the attending physician advised her that without mitral valve replacement she would die within days. She refused the operation which prompted the physician to call in a psychiatrist. He concluded that she had a personality disorder, and although frightened of dying, she was probably more frightened of the surgery. It was at this point that the issue of competence arose. Although both the psychiatrist and treating physician believed the patient understood the consequences of her refusal to have the surgery, they felt that she could be declared incompetent.

Surgery was performed, the patient survived and voluntarily agreed to a second operation a few months later when the replacement valve failed.

In this case the physicians, by questioning the decision made by the patient, in effect questioning her autonomy, actually saved her life.

Questions to consider for discussion

1. Was the attending physician right to call in the psychiatrist for a consultation in this case?

2. From an ethical perspective, what is to be said about the actions of the psychiatrist? Should the valve replacement surgery have been performed?

References

Chouinard, A. 1988. Bioethics in the critical care unit: "Damned if you do and damned if you don't." *Canadian Medical Association Journal* 139:1180-1182.

Kleinman, I. 1991. The right to refuse treatment: Ethical considerations for the competent patient. *Canadian Medical Association Journal* 144:1219-1222.

CASE 9.3
Anencephalic Babies as Organ Donors

Anencephalic babies are infants born without the part of their brain that makes thought, sight, communication and feeling possible. These are the very qualities, many would aver, that make us human beings. More than half of these children die within a day of birth, and 90% are dead within one week. Everyone in the medical community knows that the expected life-span of live-born anencephalics is very short. Yet the potential exists for some good to come out of these unfortunate situations if the anencephalics' healthy organs could be transplanted into needy recipients.

In October 1987, a young male child was born with a fatal heart defect. That newborn's sole hope for survival was a transplant. The only possible donor was an infant of his size. Three hours after birth, a transplant was performed with the donor heart taken from an anencephalic girl. The transplant operation, the first on such a young patient, was successful; a young child was given a second chance to live. (L. Cohen, "An ethics committee's ethical dilemma." *Western Report* 4(1), Jan. 23, 1989, p.23). This case raised a host of ethical issues and provoked widespread discussion.

Prior to posing some ethical questions that arise from this case, some general ethical concerns will be raised. These will serve as a more comprehensive basis for the moral discourse prompted by the specific issue.

Questions to consider for discussion

1. Should anencephalic newborns ever be considered as potential organ donors?

2. Is it possible to justify the use of aggressive life-support measures to sustain anencephalics in anticipation of brain death and a tissue-matched recipient coming together within a reasonable time frame?

3. Should anencephalics be regarded as true persons?

4. Should the legal definitions of death, particularly brain death, be revised for such patients?

   SPECIFIC ISSUE. In this case one question will likely provoke sufficient discussion of many of the ethical issues involved.

5. From an ethical perspective, were the physicians right in using the heart of an anencephalic infant as a donor organ for another baby?

Reference

Cohen, L. 1989. An ethics committee's ethical dilemma. *Western Report.* 4 (1):23

CASE 9.4
Alternative Therapy

In the fall of 1994, the Alberta College of Physicians and Surgeons (ACPS) was actively investigating six physicians for practicing chelation therapy, a medical procedure banned in that province. Chelation therapy involves the intravenous use of ethylenediamintetraacetic acid. Those physicians who believe in the procedure claim that the treatment removes plaque and reverses hardening of the arteries. Chelation therapy is an approved procedure for treating patients who have toxic metal poisoning but, according to the ACPS, it is unproven for cardiac cases and, as such, has been banned for use in such situations.

Interest in chelation therapy has increased considerably in the past few years. In late October 1994, the Chelation Therapy Society of Alberta had more than 1,500 registered members. In countries such as New Zealand, Australia, Germany and the rest of Europe, chelation therapy is accepted as being of benefit to some cardiac patients.

Apparently the action of the ACPS was initiated from within the College, since it appears that no patient complaints were cited.

Chelation therapy is sometimes categorized under the heading of alternative medicine, and some observers see the action of the ACPS as an attempt to maintain control over all medical practice within the province.

Questions to consider for discussion

1. Since the procedure has been approved in other countries and, if not actually effecting a cure, chelation therapy causes no harm, from an ethical perspective is it right for the ACPS to be investigating its own member physicians who are utilizing this therapy?

2. What ethical assessment can be rendered on the physicians who are using a non-approved therapy on their patients?

3. Does the fact that a patient requests chelation therapy modify the moral judgment rendered?

References

Breckenridge, J., and D. Saunders. 1995. Bitter medicine. *The Globe and Mail*. June 3, D1, D5.

Lowry, M. 1994. Bad medicine? *The Calgary Herald*. Sept. 3, B6.

Walker, R. 1994. Alberta college investigating six MDs for practicing chelation therapy. *Medical Post*. Oct. 25, p.12.

_____. 1995. Alternative therapies may soon get nod. *The Calgary Herald*. Oct. 6, A4.

CASE 9.5
Placebos

Standard operating procedure to test a new medication involves using a double-blind experiment. From a scientific perspective, this process is required to ensure objective results. Half the patients in the study are administered the new drug, while the other half are given a placebo, a pill that looks the same as the actual medication but is basically an innocuous substance such as sugar. Even the physicians and nurses who are part of the study do not know which patients are receiving the actual medication and which patients are receiving the placebos.

S.D., a patient in an Ottawa hospital, who had part of his fingers amputated due to circulatory problems, accused the hospital staff of substituting placebos at times in place of medication to relieve his pain. So severe was his pain that he locked himself in the bathroom and wept. S.D. felt something was amiss when the injections relieved his pain on certain days but did nothing on other days. When he complained to nurses of his severe pain, he was told by them that he needed to wait until the next scheduled (morphine) injection.

Two weeks after he was released from the hospital, S.D. was contacted by a hospital official who stated that there had been some problems with his medication.

A spokeswoman from the Ontario Nurses Association (ONA) admitted that two nurses, one male and the other female, had been fired by the hospital in question for injecting the patient with a placebo instead of morphine. Further details were unavailable because the firings were being appealed by the ONA.

S.D. has hired a lawyer to sue the hospital. His lawyer maintains that S.D. was told that he was receiving morphine but, since he is a recovering drug addict, it was not working. S.D. admits to having been hooked on heroin for many years, but at the time of his surgery, he was clean. (J. Elliott, Hospital gave placebo for pain, man says. *The Ottawa Citizen*, June 21, 1996, C1, C2).

Questions to consider for discussion

1. Ethically speaking, is it right for physicians to involve patients in experiments without first obtaining their consent?

2. Was it right for the nurses to have injected the patient with a placebo when it was obvious he was in severe pain?

3. On the assumption that the nurses were instructed by a physician (in most cases the only person authorized to prescribe morphine), is it ethically defensible to claim that they had no alternative but to follow the orders?

4. From an ethical perspective, what moral judgment can be rendered on the administrators of the hospital who condoned this practice?

Reference

Elliott, J. 1996. Hospital gave placebo for pain, man says. *The Ottawa Citizen*, June 21, C1, C2.

CASE 9.6
Experimental Procedure

AIDS patient J.G. had had most of his immune system destroyed by the HIV virus. Because of his desperate medical condition, his physicians decided radical action was required. Permission was obtained from the Food and Drug Administration (FDA) to transplant baboon marrow into the patient. Since baboons are immune to HIV, J.G.'s physicians hoped the animal's disease-fighting cells would take root. If that actually happened, the patient might survive. It would be months before a determination could be made about the efficacy of the treatment.

Transplanting baboon bone marrow into a human patient poses a number of potential risks for persons other than the patient because of the numerous pathogens that baboons carry. People could become infected with illnesses not seen before in human beings. These concerns apparently prompted a doctors' group, the Physicians Committee for Responsible Medicine, to ask U.S. federal investigators in the Office for Protection from Research Risks to determine if the transplant of baboon bone marrow into an AIDS patient could endanger the public.

In defending the approval granted, the FDA acknowledged that there were risks, but they believed that enough precautions had been taken to justify the safety of the experiment. Indeed, the FDA asserted that prior to giving approval additional precautions were ordered to make the experiment safer.

Approval was granted even though the government agency developing guidelines for animal-to-human transplants (to prevent the spread of new infectious diseases) had not completed its work at that time, near the end of December 1995.

A number of ethical issues emerges from this scenario (*The Globe and Mail*, Dec. 19, 1995, A13) and the behavior of a number of individuals needs to be assessed.

Questions to consider for discussion

Based on the information provided it is reasonable to conclude that the procedure undertaken, transplanting baboon bone marrow into a human being, falls under the category of experimenting with human beings.

1. What ethical judgment can be rendered on J.G.'s physicians for using this untested procedure?

2. Assuming that J.G.'s physicians knew that guidelines for animal-to-human transplants were in the development stage but not yet finalized, was it ethical for them to request permission to transplant baboon bone marrow into their patient?

3. Obviously the officials in the FDA were aware that the guidelines for animal-to-human transplants were not complete. In light of this knowledge, how ethical was it for them to approve the treatment even though they had demanded more safeguards be used in the experiment?

4. Once permission was granted by the FDA, how ethical was it for the Physicians Committee for Responsible Medicine to request the federal Office for Protection from Research Risks to investigate the dangers to the public?

Reference

Associated Press. 1995. MDs urge probe of baboon marrow transplant. *The Globe and Mail*, Dec. 19, A13.

CASE 9.7
Penalizing a Physician

The College of Physicians and Surgeons of Ontario found Dr. L.B., an Ottawa psychiatrist, guilty of dishonorable and unprofessional conduct (E. Medline, Lawyer wants doctor's penalty kept secret. *The Ottawa Citizen*, June 29, 1996, C1). He was charged and convicted of attempting to seduce the mother of a young patient he had been treating. In a telephone call to the woman, Dr. L.B. made "inappropriate" and "offensive" comments, including a suggestion that she take a trip with him to a country in the South Pacific.

Following the hearing, Dr. L.B. was allowed to continue practicing until his penalty hearing, which was held in June 1996. At that hearing, Dr. L.B.'s lawyer made a plea that the penalty imposed be kept secret to avoid sensational media coverage. To support the request, the lawyer voiced concern that the focus of the media reports would be on "the salacious aspects of the case" which would, in his view, offer a distorted picture of the physician's conduct.

The article detailing the current situation also included a statement about an earlier, unrelated case, where Dr. L.B. had been found guilty of having sex with a patient and was suspended for three months.

Representatives from the media and a concerned citizens group stated that the public has a right to know what penalties are imposed on physicians for misconduct as physicians are in a position of trust.

Questions to consider for discussion

1. What ethical assessment can be rendered on the lawyer for even requesting that the penalty be kept secret?

2. What ethical assessment can be rendered on Dr. L.B. for allowing his lawyer to make the request for secrecy?

3. From a moral perspective, was it right for *The Ottawa Citizen* to include comments about a previous suspension for improper conduct by Dr. L.B. in their report of the current case?

Reference

Medline, E. 1996. Lawyer wants doctor's penalty kept secret. *The Ottawa Citizen*, June 29, C1.

CASE 9.8

Physicians, Pharmaceutical Companies and Gifts

Many of the physicians who traveled to attend the annual meeting of the American Academy of Dermatology "enjoyed accommodations, dinners and entertainment paid for by drug companies" (Chrenn et al., 1989, p.3448). Senior residents in one training program each received a cheque for $156, presumably to defray transportation costs, from a pharmaceutical company whose representative took the opportunity to extol the merits of one of their products. This scenario is not unique; it can be found at the annual meetings of all medical specialists and at other medical conferences. Drug companies use a wide variety of means and spend considerable sums of money on marketing and advertising their products. Such efforts are not confined to annual meetings and medical conferences.

One physician, testifying at a recent U.S. Senate Labor Committee hearing, listed the following items he received as gifts and gimmicks to remind him to use a specific drug: "golf balls with a company or drug logo, rulers, pens, pencils, note pads, mugs, glasses, cups, hats, caps, shirts, magnets, towels, tie tacks, clipboards, a large variety of anatomic models, games, puzzles, socks, visors, packages of candy, gum, popcorn, tickets to shows, dinners, weekend getaways, golf fees, tennis balls and cash" (McLeod, 1991, p.4). Senator Edward M. Kennedy, chairman of the Committee conducting the hearing, in commenting on the estimated $5 billion a year the drug industry spends on promotion in the United States alone, stated that "much of the spending is legitimate and in the public interest ... but some is not" (McLeod, 1991, p.4). Since marketing and advertising expenditures drive up the retail price of drugs, people beset by illness are compelled to pay high costs for their prescriptions.

Pharmaceutical companies and other corporations who serve the medical community are rendering an important service in spending money on educating physicians about their newest products. Physicians apprised of the newest medical developments are in a position to offer their patients state-of-the art treatment. It is also accurate to state that companies promote their products as a means to increase sales and profits. Profits, in part, are used to finance research, which should result in further advances in medical treatment.

Gift giving by pharmaceutical companies has escalated in the recent past (Rowlins, 1984). One drug company set up a frequent-flyer-type plan for physicians who prescribed one of its products. After fifty prescriptions, the participating doctor was given a free airline ticket to any destination in the continental United States (McLeod, 1991, p.4). Under the guise of participation in a "study," doctors were offered a $1,200 grant-in-aid for answering "a few simple questions about patients receiving an expensive drug" (McLeod, 1991, p.4).

Companies host dinners for physicians at the finest restaurants or hotels and, at times, even present honoraria of $100 or $200 to each doctor attending just for listening to a presentation about the sponsor's product. Most lavish are the free vacations for physicians and their spouses in such places as Hawaii and the Caribbean, generally scheduled during the winter months. Physicians may attend one or two lectures to learn more about the host company's products but the rest of the time is spent on recreational activities. Attending these lectures satisfies the requirements of some state certification boards for participation in continuing education programs. This supposed educational component provides a handy rationale for the drug companies; it enables them to claim that they are contributing to the ongoing education of physicians. In one sense it can be claimed that everyone benefits from this arrangement.

Acceptance of gifts from drug companies or other corporations that serve the medical community carries with it certain consequences. As noted above, the cost for these promotions is factored into the eventual price paid by the patient. Once a gift is accepted, a certain relationship is established between the donor and the recipient; an obligation, even if only minimal or vague, has been incurred by the person accepting what has been proffered. Once that obligation has been incurred, a subtle influence may be at work which raises a range of ethical issues.

Questions to consider for discussion

1. Will physicians be more inclined to prescribe a particular drug even if it is very expensive?

2. Will the physician put selfish interests ahead of those of the patient's in order to fulfill an implicit obligation incurred when a gift was accepted?

3. From an ethical perspective, is it ever right for a pharmaceutical company or any other corporation serving the medical community to give gifts to physicians and surgeons?

4. Is there a difference between education, advertising and marketing? Which of these, if any, can corporations use ethically when dealing with the medical community?

5. Is it ethical for a physician or surgeon to accept any gift from one of these companies? Which sort of gifts and/or marketing gimmicks are ethically acceptable and which are not?

References

Bricker, E.M. 1989. Industrial marketing and medical ethics. *New England Journal of Medicine* 320:1690-1692.

Chrenn, M.M., S. Landefeld, and T.H. Murray. 1989. Doctors, drug companies, and gifts. *Journal of the American Medical Association* 262:3448-3451.

Fisher, D.S. 1992. Observations on ethical problems and terminal care. *Yale Journal of Biology and Medicine* 65:105-120.

McLeod, D. 1991. Drug firms' payola practice under fire. *AARP Bulletin* 32(2):4.

Rawlins, M.D. 1984. Doctors and the drug makers. *Lancet* ii:276-278.

CASE 9.9
Physician as Finder for a Fee

In many areas of business, finder's fees are an accepted and acceptable procedure. These rewards or commissions are regarded as compensation for services rendered. A real estate agent refers a customer to a bank that has a specific investment instrument and is paid a modest fee by the bank once the deal is made. This is one example of someone receiving a finder's fee. Another example would be an insurance agent referring a client to an antique shop after hearing the client express a desire to purchase a specific product. After the item is purchased, the store sends the agent a finder's fee. In the business world, such incidents generally do not provoke ethical questions. Does the same line of thinking apply to finder's fees in medicine?

Clinical studies, using human subjects, are often required to test new drugs, new equipment, or innovative medical procedures in order to determine their efficacy and/or safety. The results of clinical studies are required in order to obtain government approval for the sale of that drug or of new equipment, or to implement the new procedure. Without favorable results from clinical studies using human subjects, regulatory bodies would be hard-pressed to grant approval except in some dire emergency. It then follows that drug companies and medical equipment manufacturers (where applicable) are anxious to have clinical tests conducted involving a sufficient number of subjects.

There has been a chronic problem in finding sufficient subjects to participate in clinical studies. Standard recruiting methods—posting public notices in places where large number of subjects will see them, presentations to groups explaining the medical and social benefits to be derived from that study, and placing ads in the media—most often do not obtain sufficient subjects. It appears that more aggressive procedures are needed to recruit sufficient numbers.

Principal Investigator Dr. A.B. experienced considerable difficulty in recruiting the required number of subjects to test a new drug that the pharmaceutical company had targeted for public sale twelve months after the date of completion of the clinical test. The drug in question was seen by the company as a major advance on what was currently available. In addition, they had heard rumors that their main competitor, Company T, was well advanced in developing a similar product. In an attempt to alleviate the situation, Dr. A.B. sent a letter to each of the residents in that specialty in that city's hospitals offering a $350 finder's fee for each patient referred who actually enrolled in the study.

Dr. L.M., a senior resident, referred three patients to Dr. A.B. All of the money Dr. L.M. received from the finder's fees ($1,050) was remitted to the bank immediately to help reduce the $35,000 debt still owing on the doctor's student loan.

Questions to consider for discussion

1. Was it right for Dr. A.B. to offer a finder's fee to residents in return for referrals to the clinical study?

2. Is it ethical for the pharmaceutical firm to supply funds to pay for finder's fees?

3. Was it right for Dr. L.M. to accept a finder's fee for referring patients to Dr. A.B.'s clinical study?

References

Bricker, E.M. 1989. Sounding board. Industrial marketing and medical ethics. *New England Journal of Medicine* 320(25):1690-1692.

Chren, M.M., C.S. Landefeld, and T.H. Murray. 1989. Doctors, drug companies, and gifts. *Journal of the American Medical Association* 262(24):3448-3451.

Lind, S.E. 1990. Sounding board. Finder's fees for research subjects. *New England Journal of Medicine* 323(3):192-194.

McLeod, D. 1991. Drug firms' payola practices under fire. *AARP Bulletin* 32(2):4-5.

Shimm, D.S., and R.G. Spence. 1991. Industry reimbursement for entering patients into clinical trials: Legal and ethical issues. *Annals of Internal Medicine* 115(2):148-151.

CASE 9.10
The Right to Die

Medical practitioners devote their professional careers to improving the health and preserving the lives of their patients. Illness and injury are seen as foes to be overcome and vanquished, so that health can be restored and life prolonged. However, there are times when a decision made by a patient directs physicians to either refrain from acting or to act in a way that is contrary to the entrenched medical ethos of preserving life. This is the situation in the following case, which is further complicated by the involvement of both legal and ethical issues that are, at times, inextricably intertwined.

A twenty-five-year-old patient, Ms. B., suffered from a nerve disorder called Guillain-Barré syndrome. This nerve disorder had left her paralyzed from the neck down and unable to breathe without the aid of a ventilator. At this advanced stage of the disease, medical science has no treatment that will effect a cure or alleviate the symptoms. It appears that all that can be done is to use a ventilator to prolong life.

Implicit in the physician-patient relationship is the consent for treatment. This implied consent may even be firmer in a hospital setting, given our understanding of the role and purpose society ascribes to this institution. After a period of more than two years, and with a prognosis of no improvement, Ms. B. asked the doctors to discontinue the ventilation, which, in effect, meant she would be allowed to die. Citing the possibility of criminal charges being laid if they complied with the request, her physicians and the hospital denied her request. Since a patient has the right to refuse treatment, this is the point at which the legal and ethical aspects intertwine.

When apprised of the refusal, Ms. B. hired a lawyer and took her case to the Quebec Superior Court. A hearing took place both in the courtroom and in the patient's hospital room. After considering all the arguments, The Honourable Mr. Justice J.D. ruled that Ms. B. "has the right to demand cessation of the respiratory support being given her" (What judge said of woman's right to die. *The Toronto*

Star, Jan. 8, 1992, A12). Citing an American judgment, Mr. Justice J.D. added, "In any event, declining life-sustaining medical treatment may not properly be viewed as suicide. Refusing medical intervention merely allows the disease to take its natural course" (A15). Included in the decision was a stipulation that, after a thirty-day appeal period, and upon renewed consent from the patient (in effect, repeating her decision to discontinue treatment), the physician would remove the ventilator and appropriate sedatives could be administered to allow her to die with dignity.

From a legal perspective, Mr. Justice J.D. noted that such actions would not be criminal as set out in the Criminal code. Mr. Justice J.D.'s ruling seems to have resolved the legal aspects of the case.

No appeals were launched. After the thirty-day period had expired, the use of the ventilator was discontinued.

Questions to consider for discussion

1. Despite the judge's legal ruling—that declining medical treatment and letting the disease take its natural course is not a criminal act—from an ethical perspective what judgment can rendered on such an act?

2. Were the physicians and the hospital right in refusing Ms. B.'s original request?

3. Was Ms. B. right in taking her physicians and the hospital to court?

4. What is the ethical status of Ms. B.'s request to have the ventilator removed?

5. Do you agree with the judge's statement that declining life-sustaining medical treatment, that is, allowing the nature of the illness (whatever that means) to run its course, may not be properly viewed as suicide?

References

Grant, A. 1993. Questions of life and death. *Canadian Nurse* 89(5):31-34.

Lavery, J. 1992. When merely staying alive is morally intolerable. *The Globe and Mail*, Jan. 7, A13.

[No Author]. 1992. What judge said of woman's right to die. *The Toronto Star*, Jan. 8, A12.

CASE 9.11

Helping to Alleviate Suffering before Death

Toward the end of November 1991, the family of patient Mr. J.S., aged seventy-eight, asked his physicians to remove him from life-support systems. Mr. S. had gone into an irreversible coma after a knee operation in one hospital and was transferred to another hospital suffering from kidney, liver and lung failure. There was consensus among the medical staff that he would not live without life-support systems. In compliance with the family's request, the attending physician had him removed from the ventilator after giving him two injections of morphine and valium to ease the pain. Mr. S. was expected to die within an hour.

A young male nurse, who had graduated only eighteen months earlier, was left alone in the room and watched the patient choke to death. As he witnessed the agony of the patient, Nurse S.M. "'became distraught' and 'in a state of emotional turmoil … without a doctor's order' administered potassium chloride to the patient, who died within minutes" (C. Mungan and G. Abbote, Sentence suspended in euthanasia case. *The Globe and Mail*, Aug. 25, 1992, A1). With the final outcome already determined, the injection of potassium chloride served to shorten the time of agony for the patient. In one sense it could be claimed that all Nurse S.M. did was expedite the final result of the process inaugurated by the physician.

Nurse S.M. informed the hospital authorities of his action when he found out that an autopsy was to be performed. Since potassium chloride is a naturally occurring substance in the body, it is unlikely that it would have been detected or implicated in the cause of death. Nurse S.M. was charged with first-degree murder; this event was viewed as a case of euthanasia.

Euthanasia, no matter how eloquently it is rationalized, results in the death of one person (or a number of people) at the hands of another person (or group of people). As such it violates an almost universally held law against taking other people's lives, which is usually seen as a foundation of all civilized societies.

At the trial and throughout the proceedings, the members of the patient's family consistently maintained that they did not want Nurse S.M. sent to jail as a result of his action.

At the trial, Nurse S.M. pleaded guilty to a lesser charge of administering a noxious substance. He was given a suspended sentence, put on probation for three years and barred from working in any health-care or geriatric facility in any capacity while on probation. He was ordered to surrender his nursing licence. Since the defense attorney had suggested the sentence, it meant that Nurse S.M. was voluntarily withdrawing from the nursing profession. A spokesperson for the hospital explained that new nurses, such as S.M., underwent a ten-week orientation program that included an examination of the non-resuscitation guidelines published by the Canadian Medical Association and the Canadian Nurses Association. She also commented that it was unusual for a nurse with such limited experience to be left alone with a dying patient.

Questions to consider for discussion

1. From an ethical perspective, what judgment can be rendered on the physician who removed the patient from the ventilator after giving him injections of morphine and valium?

2. What ethical judgment can be rendered on the physician for leaving the patient in the care of a nurse until death occurred?

3. Ethically, should the physician have been responsible for selecting the nurse who would stay with the patient in his final hour of life?

4. What ethical judgment can be rendered on the hospital administration for allowing a nurse to be the only medical practitioner present during the patient's final hour of life?

5. Given the situation described, what ethical judgment can be rendered on the nursing supervisor for assigning a nurse with such limited experience to this case?

6. Within the context of the decision made by the patient's family and the action of the physician in administering morphine and valium and then removing the ventilator, was the nurse right in taking action to end the patient's agony?

Reference

Mungan, C., and G. Abbate. 1992. Sentence suspended in euthanasia case. *The Globe and Mail*, Aug. 25, A1, A12.

CASE 9.12
Rent-a-Womb

Bob and Nancy, a childless Canadian couple, have experienced the full impact of infertility for ten years of married life. They have tried everything from fertility drugs to private adoption without success. When it was finally determined that Linda was infertile, they turned to surrogacy. Bob's sperm was artificially inseminated into the surrogate mother while she was taking fertility drugs to increase the likelihood of pregnancy. This procedure was done in California through a private agency that made all the necessary arrangements.

Costs involved totaled just over $55,000. Approximately half of that sum was paid to the surrogate mother. Some fees were disbursed to doctors, psychologists and lawyers affiliated with the agency, and the agency's fee for the transaction was slightly more than $23,000. There are no such agencies in Canada, where it is illegal for any woman to receive "consideration" for carrying someone else's baby.

Bob and Nancy were more than pleased with the results of the first effort. A little girl, the biological offspring of Bob (since his sperm was used) and the surrogate mother, was born. To complete the process, from a legal perspective, Nancy was required to adopt the baby. Adoption was effected in the United States since it is easier to do there than in Canada where the law prohibits money being exchanged for the child.

After the birth, Bob and Nancy vowed to maintain contact with the surrogate mother and her husband. They also proclaimed publicly their intention to explain to their daughter the unusual circumstances surrounding her birth when she became old enough to understand and appreciate the situation. She, most likely, would be different in this respect from all of her friends.

When asked about receiving payment for carrying the baby, the surrogate mother replied that she would have borne Bob and Nancy's baby for free but the agency involved has a policy which states that women should be compensated for what they do. She then added that because her own family was complete—she and her husband have three of their own children—she had no qualms about surrendering the baby. She claimed to have no maternal instincts toward this baby, because she knew from the start that the child was Bob and Nancy's, not hers.

Because the first venture turned out so well, Bob and Nancy opted for a second child in the same manner, with the same surrogate mother, once their daughter reached two and one-half years of age. In the interim the costs had risen to almost $70,000. The surrogate mother affirmed that she would always love both children because they were a part of her, but she also added that they were not hers because they were not created by her with her husband.

Artificial insemination, in this case the sperm from a married man inseminated into a woman who is not his wife, is a medical procedure designed to produce a fetus without adultery occurring.

Questions to consider for discussion

1. Is adultery truly averted by the use of artificial insemination?

2. Is childlessness an illness that requires medical attention? Should community medical resources be devoted to this condition?

3. From an ethical perspective, were Bob and Nancy right in selecting surrogacy as a means to end their childlessness?

4. Were they right to seek out an agency in California knowing that Canadian law forbids payment to surrogate mothers or money changing hands during adoption?

5. Is it ever right for a woman to be a surrogate mother?

6. The event described in this case study can be regarded as establishing a two-tiered medical system for a particular component of medicine. If a couple can afford the costs involved they can then have/obtain a baby through surrogacy, but if they do not have the funds, that option is unavailable. From a social ethical perspective, is that fair?

Reference

Moysa, M. 1996. Couple pays high price to surrogate for priceless child. *The Ottawa Citizen*, July 16, A1, A2.

CASE 9.13
Abort One Twin

A single, twenty-eight-year-old British mother of one child, sixteen weeks pregnant with twins, instructed her gynecologist to abort one fetus. Since she is unmarried, her tight financial straits, she claimed, could be stretched to cover the expenses of only one additional child, but not two.

When the gynecologist expressed serious reservations about complying with the request, the woman told him she would rather abort both fetuses than give birth to twins. Faced with that scenario, the gynecologist, after consulting with medical colleagues, concluded that it would be preferable to terminate one pregnancy as soon as possible and leave one alive, rather than lose two babies (H. Branswell, Woman's plan to abort one twin sparks uproar. *The Ottawa Citizen*, Aug. 6, 1996, A1).

A spokesperson from the British Medical Association (head of the ethics committee) commented that, from an ethical perspective, this case was like any other abortion. Contrary views were expressed that focused on the mother's decision which, in effect, chose life for one fetus and death for the other. Additional questions were posed about what the mother would tell the surviving twin when he or she had grown up and how the mother would cope with the knowledge that she had chosen to abort one twin because the living twin would be a constant reminder of the choice she made.

And how was that child going to feel?

When news of the impending abortion became public, many pro-life organizations spoke out against the decision. A number of these groups offered considerable sums of money to avert the abortion; sufficient funds were pledged to ensure that the family would have enough money for their needs. When apprised of the offers, the gynecologist maintained he would not advise his patient of them, since, in his view, that would be a breach of physician-patient confidentiality. Further probing revealed that the abortion had already been performed, and now questions were being raised about breaches of physician-patient confidentiality, because it appears that it was the patient's gynecologist who made the details of the case public.

Selective termination was used to abort one fetus. Selective termination is the name given to a medical procedure where one fetus in a multiple pregnancy is killed by inserting a needle into it. What remains shrivels in the uterus and is passed from the womb when the surviving twin is born. Selective termination is generally done when one fetus suffers abnormalities or when several embryos develop during infertility treatment, thus imperiling the chances of the mother giving birth. It appears that this was the first known case in Britain that involved healthy twin fetuses.

Questions to consider for discussion

1. From an ethical perspective, was the mother right, given her financial limitations, to request the abortion of one fetus?

2. Was the gynecologist right in complying with the patient's request to abort one fetus even when threatened (blackmailed) with the ominous prospect of having both fetuses aborted?

3. What is the ethical status of the attempts made by the anti-abortion groups to intervene in this case? Isn't this matter something between a physician and patient?

4. Was the gynecologist right in making the details of this case public?

5. From an ethical perspective, is this case just like any other abortion?

Reference

Branwell, H. 1996. Woman's plan to abort one twin sparks uproar. *The Ottawa Citizen*, August 6, A1.

CASE 9.14
Abort Some/Many Fetuses

A few days after the furor caused by the decision of the pregnant mother of one child to abort one of the twins she was carrying (CASE 9.13—Abort One Twin), another pregnancy and abortion incident emerged in the same country. Since this case—details are provided below—is, in one sense, contrary to the previous one, it invites us to examine the ethical issues involved from a different perspective.

M.A., a thirty-one-year-old woman who already had one child, was involved in a fertility program to help her to conceive again. When she did become pregnant, her physician informed her that she was carrying eight fetuses. This condition obviously required special care, so she was referred to a specialist. Two prominent gynecologists were in agreement "that the chances of all eight babies being born alive was 'extremely remote'" (M. Weaver, Woman carrying eight fetuses risks health of self and babies. *The Ottawa Citizen*, Aug. 10, 1996, A10; Octuplet mother pledges to have all her babies. *The Ottawa Citizen*, Aug. 11, 1996, A2). Continuing with the pregnancies posed a serious risk to the mother's health and greatly increased the likelihood of a miscarriage and very premature labor. Selective termination of a number of the fetuses was recommended.

Dr. Peter Bromich, one of the prominent gynecologists, is quoted as saying, "The biggest single cause of handicapped babies is being born too early or having too many babies in the womb" (*The Ottawa Citizen*, A10). Handicapped babies drain community resources for as long as they live.

The medical advice given, for the benefit of the mother, for the benefit of her unborn children, and for the benefit of society was to reduce the number of fetuses so that the odds of a normal birth for the remaining fetuses would greatly increase. M.A.'s physician, Prof. Kypros Nicolaides, was quoted as saying "that if she continued with the pregnancy she would end up with no babies, whereas an embryo reduction would give her a chance of saving some of them" (*The Ottawa Citizen*, A2).

Despite this medical advice, the expectant mother announced that she would go ahead with her pregnancy. "I want nature to take its course" the mother is quoted as saying (Woman pregnant with 8 rejects abortion advice. *The Toronto Star*, Aug. 11, 1996, A5). Anti-abortion groups welcomed the news that M.A. had refused fetus reduction. Given the publicity generated by this case, it seems safe to assume that everyone was aware of the severe risks to all eight fetuses. Despite this, "Professor Jack Scarisbrick of the anti-abortion group Life told *The News of the World:* 'I am delighted by her pro-life response to this challenge. It's wonderful news'" *(The Toronto Star,* Aug. 11, op. cit.).

M.A. and her boyfriend, P.H., hired a publicist, who negotiated a contract for them with the British newspaper *The News of the World.* M.A. would earn money from her pregnancy by selling her story to the newspaper. However, "the amount of money she will make from selling her story depends on the number of babies she bears (Potential mother of 8 to be paid per live baby. *The Ottawa Citizen*, Aug. 12, 1996, A6). M.A. and P.H. would receive reduced payment from *The News of the World* if any of the eight fetuses died. Payment, on a sliding scale, would vary according to the number of babies born. The publicist attributed the financial arrangement to "market forces."

According to the publicist, the mother's decision to "allow nature to take its course," that is, to reject selective termination, was not affected by the newspaper deal.

Questions to consider for discussion

1. What ethical judgment can be rendered on the two prominent physicians who recommended selective termination of a number of the fetuses?

2. After receiving the advice and recommendation of the two prominent physicians who advocated selective termination, what ethical judgment can be rendered on the mother for refusing?

3. What is the ethical status of the newspaper *The News of the World* for paying the mother for the rights to her story?

4. What can be said, ethically, about the contract which will pay the mother according to the number of live births?

5. Given the medical pronouncement of the threat to all eight fetuses and the threat to the health of the mother, what ethical judgment can be rendered on the spokesman for the anti-abortion group Life, who expressed delight at the mother's refusal of selective termination?

References

Weaver, M. 1996. Woman carrying eight fetuses risks health of self and babies. *The Ottawa Citizen, Aug. 10, A11.*

[No Author]. 1996. Octuplet mother pledges to have all her babies. *The Ottawa Citizen, Aug. 11, A2.*

[No Author]. 1996. Woman pregnant with 8 requests abortion advice. *The Toronto Star*, Aug. 11, A5.

[No Author], 1996. Potential mother of 8 to be paid per live baby. *The Ottawa Citizen*, Aug. 12, A6.

CASE 9.15

Demand for Continuing Futile Therapy

A sixty-eight-year-old retired businessman with severe emphysema was admitted to hospital with progressive shortness of breath. He had a left lower lobe pneumonia and treatment, consisting of bronchodilation and antibiotics, was started immediately. He initially stabilized, even improved slightly, but subsequently fatigued and had worsening dyspnea. His request for mechanical ventilation to help him breathe resulted in a transfer to the ICU, where he was provided with assisted mechanical ventilation. After twelve days, efforts to wean him from the ventilator were proving unsuccessful, despite the clearing of his pneumonia.

This patient had been hospitalized on many occasions in the past and had been on a mechanical ventilator twice previously for similar episodes, but had not been in the ICU for the same lengthy period. When discharged, he was virtually housebound and needed continuous oxygen to help him breathe. His activities were severely limited, consisting mainly of watching television and receiving visits from his grandchildren.

In the ICU, a tracheotomy was performed to enable continued mechanical ventilation. Efforts to strengthen his respiratory muscles were slowed by cardiac arrhythmias. Light sedation kept him relatively comfortable and alert. His physician, in consultation with three other specialists, concluded that additional therapy to improve his condition would be of no value.

After twenty-five days in the ICU, a facility that was becoming overcrowded due to the presence of other severely ill patients, the patient was approached by his physician regarding further therapy. The patient was told that his lungs were too involved with emphysema to ever allow him to breathe without support. Unfortunately, no long-term facility existed locally which provided this type of care. One final trial of weaning was recommended and, if unsuccessful, a withdrawal of extraordinary support was recommended.

In response, the patient and his wife demanded the continued use of the ventilator and insisted that everything be done to help improve the condition of the patient.

Questions to consider for discussion

1. Are physicians, even the most experienced and sophisticated specialists, ever ethically justified in stating that no further therapy will be helpful?

2. What ethical judgment can be rendered on the physician's decision to recommend a final trial of weaning training and, if unsuccessful, the withdrawal of extraordinary support?

3. From a medical perspective, is it fair to other very sick people to have one patient occupy a bed in the ICU for twenty-five days?

4. Ethically, was this patient right in demanding continued use of limited resources (ICU, ventilator) when the potential healing benefit is minimal or even zero?

CASE 9.16
Full Disclosure: Whose Responsibility?

A sixty-year-old recently retired civil servant has been diagnosed as having right upper lobe adenocarcinoma of the lung. Further examination revealed that it has already spread to the regional lymph nodes as well as the liver. He has underlying diabetes melitis and the onset of emphysema. He is referred to an oncologist for further assessment and treatment.

A range of therapies was considered, including chemotherapy, radiotherapy and palliative therapy. The chemotherapist is a fairly young, very aggressive physician, who regards each case as a personal challenge. In this case he tells the patient that there was a 70% response rate among former patients he has treated who displayed similar symptoms. He has had considerable experience with similar drug combinations and indicated to the patient that he should be able to tolerate the treatment fairly well. Very little information is conveyed to the patient by the chemotherapist about the potential range and significance of the side effects. At the conclusion of the interview, the chemotherapist recommends an early start for the treatment, noting that the sooner the intervention begins the better the chances of success. The patient agrees to start as soon as the chemotherapist can arrange an appointment.

The patient and his wife, who are medically naive, leave the chemotherapist's office feeling fairly optimistic. They then visit their family physician who listens carefully to the details of their visit with the chemotherapist. The family physician wonders why there was almost no mention made of the potential side effects and questions how enlightened the patient was when he consented to the chemotherapy, but says nothing. Far better, he thinks, to have an optimistic patient at the start of treatment than a pessimistic one, since he is convinced that a patient's attitude is an important factor in the healing process.

Nothing is said to the patient by the family physician, who also refrains from commenting to the chemotherapist about his professional conduct in not providing more comprehensive details to enable the patient to make a better-informed decision.

Questions to consider for discussion

1. On the assumption that an optimistic attitude does have a positive impact on the healing process, was the chemotherapist ethically justified in "glossing over" the potential side effects?

2. From an ethical perspective, how much information should a physician be required to transmit to a patient so that everyone can claim there were sufficient grounds for granting informed consent?

3. After being informed by the patient about what had transpired in the chemotherapist's office, did the family physician behave ethically by not mentioning the likelihood of major side effects?

4. From the perspective of collegiality (members of the same profession) and common ethical behavior, was it right for the family physician to refrain from raising the matter of insufficient information conveyed to the patient directly with the chemotherapist?

CASE 9.17

Physician, Please Remain Silent (I)

A fifty-three-year-old married father of three teenagers is admitted to hospital with bilateral pneumonia. The initial diagnosis is atypical pneumonia and appropriate antibiotics are started. Despite the therapy, the chest x-rays reveal a worsening condition and an increasing need for oxygen is noted. Because the level of oxygenation continues to fall, the patient is moved to the ICU for assisted mechanical ventilation.

Once insulated and ventilated, a flexible bronchoscopy is performed to obtain material. Special tests conducted reveal that pneumocystis carinii is present. This pneumonia is associated with immunocomprimise and often HIV infection.

A review of the admitting history yields no risk factors for HIV infection. Physicians approach this severely ill man to inquire further about additional possible risk factors. He is able to communicate in writing, reluctantly admitting to several homosexual liaisons. Thoroughly embarrassed, and now realizing the nature and gravity of his illness, he extracts a "death bed" promise from the physician not to reveal this part of his past, and the true cause of death, to his family.

Questions to consider for discussion

1. From an ethical perspective, was it fair for the physicians to approach a critically ill patient to press for the disclosure of this aspect of his life?

2. Was the patient right in demanding that the physician refrain from telling the members of his family the real story, given the risks involved?

3. Did the physician behave ethically in agreeing to keep the information from the family?

4. From an ethical perspective, could the physician have refused the dying man's request? Should he have?

CASE 9.18

Physician, Please Remain Silent (II)

In certain ethnic communities in Canada it is commonly believed that patients should be told as little as possible about their illnesses, especially if it is serious. It is believed that bad news delivered by a physician could devastate the patient even before treatment is started.

A seventy-six-year-old retired Italian-Canadian mason presents with hemoptysis. An x-ray he brought along with him reveals a tumor. His family is present during the taking of the history, often answering the questions posed by the physician when the patient is unable to or cannot recall. When the patient goes to the examining room to change, the son and daughter plead that their father not be told if the diagnosis is cancer. They fear "it could kill him" to learn of such bad news.

This is not the first time that Dr. H. has heard this kind of request. It poses a dilemma for him: should he acknowledge the ethnic difference and keep the information from the patient, or should he follow his regular procedure and inform the patient of the true nature of his illness? Since a reply needs to be given almost instantaneously, there is no time to cogitate the pros and cons of both alternatives. As he has done in the past, Dr. H. accedes to the family's request.

Unfortunately, a malignant tumor is diagnosed, one requiring surgery. The elderly patient is not told that he has cancer in respect of the agreement made with the ever-present attentive family. The tumor subsequently recurs and radiation therapy is prescribed. Dr. H. is bothered about informed consent throughout the twenty-six month duration of the illness.

Questions to consider for discussion

1. From an ethical perspective, was it fair for the members of the patient's family to ask Dr. H. not to divulge the details of the illness to their father?

2. In a pluralistic society, was Dr. H. right in deciding to honor the wishes of the children of his patient?

3. Did Dr. H. breach the physician-patient relationship in this case?

CASE 9.19

Surrogate Motherhood: Where Is the Boundary?

In Italy there is no legal ban on surrogate motherhood, but the Italian medical body's professional code of conduct forbids it.

A thirty-five-year-old Italian woman, Angela, the mother of two children, ages eight and ten, told the news media "that she is acting as a surrogate mother and expecting two boys in a pregnancy involving five people" (Reuters, Surrogate mother carries twins from separate donors. *The Ottawa Citizen*, Mar. 8, 1997, A19). Gynecologist Pasquale Bilotta admitted that "he implanted two eggs from different women and fertilized by separate men in the surrogate mother.... Both female donors were Italian" (A19). To circumvent the Italian medical body's ban, the procedure was conducted in Switzerland where, apparently, there is no legal or medical body prohibition.

A number of commentators exclaimed that a boundary had been crossed. As one newspaper, *La Stampa*, pointed out, "Two children are being born as the offspring of five adults, of two fathers and three mothers. Here the whole concept of the family, of brothers and of twins has been blown apart" (A19). Profound questions of family kinship were raised. What, if any, would be the relationship between the two baby boys gestating within the surrogate mother? Were they twins? How could they be twins if each one is the product and/or offspring of a different couple? However, if they were both being carried by the same "mother," did that not, by our current definition and understanding of the term, make them twins?

Angela, the surrogate mother, stated that she had decided to help two childless women out of love and was not receiving any fees; she was only being reimbursed for her expenses. She is quoted as saying, "It is an act of humanity" (A19), and added that she did not want to see the babies after they were born nor did she want any information about the two couples whose babies she was carrying.

Finding women to act as surrogate mothers is difficult, yet this procedure may be the only one through which some couples can have their "own" children. It could be argued that Angela was performing a good deed which would be of great benefit to two couples who, otherwise, could not have children of their own.

Although the procedure was performed in Switzerland, this may not absolve Dr. Bilotta from blame. In the view of Aldo Pagni, president of Italy's medical order, Dr. Bilotta should face sanctions.

Questions to consider for discussion

1. Did Dr. Bilotta behave in an ethical manner by conducting the procedure in Switzerland where, apparently, it is neither against the law nor contrary to the rules of the medical association in that jurisdiction?

2. Does Italy's medical order have jurisdiction over Dr. Bilotta in this case? Can they sanction him?

3. Should they sanction him?

4. From an ethical perspective, what judgment can be rendered on Angela for (1) agreeing to carry two fetuses from two different mothers, and (2) making a decision not to see the babies after their birth?

5. After the babies are born, will she be able to maintain her resolve not to see them?

6. Was an ethical boundary crossed?

Reference

Reuters. 1997. Surrogate mother carries twins from separate donors. *The Ottawa Citizen*, Mar. 8, A19.

CASE 9.20
Faith and Healing?

Dr. C. is employed by Metropolitan Hospital. She is twenty-seven years old and a graduate from one of the country's leading medical schools. Her academic record is impressive, as she had already completed an M.Sc. in physiology prior to entering medical school and had won the University President's Medal for outstanding achievement in research. Her goal is eventually to be a researcher in the realm of neurophysiology (she has been offered several faculty positions already), but she wants first to understand the realm of medicine from the "trenches" before moving to the research laboratory. Dr. C. is a very bright, pragmatic, independent and ambitious doctor with a promising career. Dr. C. is married and has a six-year old son; her husband is a part-time consultant-writer who is able to be a stay-at-home father.

Metropolitan Hospital is a large facility located in the center of the city. It has an excellent reputation both nationally and internationally for its innovative practices in surgery and administration. The administrative staff is very progressive and makes a concerted effort to let the doctors and nurses do their job with minimal interference.

One day in October, a child of six was brought into the Emergency Room with a severe dislocation and fracture of the left tibia and medial malleolus, the result of a bad fall (and an unfortunate landing) from a play structure at school. The school attempted to contact the parents of the child immediately but were unable to until well after a decision had been made to take him to Metropolitan by ambulance. Once contacted, the parents of the boy were extremely upset that he had been taken to hospital for they were members of the Church of Christ, Scientists. The adherents of this religion do not believe in contemporary medicine; instead faith is placed in God, and prayers alone would cure all pathologies.

The parents arrived at the hospital after the boy had been admitted by the school's vice-principal, Ms. S. The boy had been prepped for immediate surgery and Dr. C. had begun the operation when the irate parents ordered her to stop at once and let them take their child to their church to be healed by the will of God. Dr. C. is not a religious person. She knew well that the surgery she was about to perform was routine, and full recovery would be probable for the boy. Without the operation, the child would never again walk with a normal gait or be able to run or to jump, as the capacity to dorsi or plantar flex and to pronate or supinate this joint would undoubtedly be permanently and severely restricted. Dr. C. was well aware of the hospital's policy that once consent has been given by a parent or guardian (i.e., by proxy), surgery can commence. Though it was not the parents who had given consent in this situation, consent nonetheless had been given by Ms. S., and Dr. C. was not about to allow this child (the same age as her son) to suffer unnecessarily a life with limited mobility. She pressed on despite the parents' demands and threats to sue.

Questions to consider for discussion

1. What individual factors are at work in this case? For the parents? For Dr. C.?

2. What values are in conflict?

3. What is the moral intensity? What factor would you use to determine intensity?

4. Does the hospital culture play a role?

5. What external variables are in conflict in this case?

Reference

Kluge, E.W. (1992). *Biomedical Ethics: In a Canadian Context*. Scarborough, Ont.: Prentice-Hall, Inc.

CASE 9.21
Cost-Benefit Ratio and Health Care

Dr. M. is the director of a health district that is given an $8.5 million annual budget by the government for organ transplantation. Each year this amount is exhausted as the demand for transplants and the availability of new technology makes a variety of procedures more readily available. Dr. M. has a Ph.D. in Health Care Administration and an M.B.A. from an American university. He has been the chief administrator for the district for the past twelve years and has experienced a number of fluctuations in the amount of dollars available for health care generally. Through all of the financial turmoil, Dr. M. has managed to keep the district in the black, a phenomenon uncommon in other health districts in the province. Dr. M.'s leadership in the health district is extremely well received. The medical and administrative staff of the seven hospitals he oversees are generally pleased with his managerial style, his fiscal responsibility and his objective style of decision making.

On June 8th, a baby boy was born and diagnosed with an irreversible heart condition. The only hope for the child's survival was a transplant. The medical staff immediately began preliminary preparation for major surgery. Dr. M. soon became aware of the child's condition and ordered a review of the hospital's budget before any further preparation was to occur. He reviewed hospital and district policies on transplant, as well as current expenditures from the transplant allocation. The facts showed that an operation of this magnitude would cost approximately $1 million to $1.4. million, and the success rate was rather low for pediatric cardiac transplants. The current allocation would be exhausted if the operation was carried out, and there remained seven months before the funds for the new budget would be received. As a consequence, the cost of this one pediatric transplant would prevent the district from performing any other transplants. The decision to operate had to be made within the next twelve hours if the boy had any chance of survival.

Questions to consider for discussion

1. Can a good, right and authentic decision be made?

2. Which ethical orientation is Dr. M. likely to employ? Why?

2. What values are in conflict?

3. Does organizational culture have a role to play? Does the health district's culture have a role to play?

4. What options are open to Dr. M.?

5. What bases can be argued for who receives a transplant? From which ethical orientation do these bases come?

CASE 9.22

Who Has the Final Right to Decide?

Baby M.R.M. was brought into the world by emergency caesarean section, fifteen weeks premature and weighing only 1 lb., 11 ozs. The infant, considered at risk of brain damage, was given a 30% to 50% chance of survival. Babies born this many weeks premature are often at risk for a wide range of other problems as well. However, recent advances in neonatology has made it possible for many infants to survive, often overcoming problems thought to be fatal a scant twenty to thirty years ago. Many actually thrive as they mature.

Prior to the delivery, the father asked the physicians at the hospital not to take any extraordinary measures to prolong his child's life. From both an ethical and a legal perspective, it is commonly accepted that parents are allowed to make medical decisions for their children, including the termination of life support. These decisions are most often made after the child has been on life support and various tests have been conducted to provide a basis for a prognosis and an evaluation of future prospects. This procedure was not followed in this case.

About an hour after the birth, the father, Dr. M, a dermatologist on staff at the same hospital, entered the neonatology ward, asked the nurses to leave and then unhooked the life-support system. An alarm sounded, which brought the medical staff back immediately, but it was too late. Shortly thereafter, the baby was pronounced dead.

Dr. P.K., the attending neonatologist, told a hospital inquiry that the baby showed signs of activity at birth and, in her professional opinion, he should be given respiratory support and diagnostic tests to assess his condition. From a medical ethical perspective the recommendation usually made is to start treatment and then, through testing, evaluate what quality of life the child and the family could expect. Following that procedure has a serious drawback; once treatment is started it is much more difficult to stop, both from an emotional and, often, a legal perspective.

In those heart-wrenching cases where a parental decision is made to terminate life support for their child it is often the physician who removes the patient from the respirator. Since Dr. M. is both the parent and a physician it could be posited that by unhooking baby M.R. from the life-support system he was merely carrying out the wishes of the parent.

Questions to Consider for Discussion

1. Does the request from one physician to another not to take extraordinary measures have a coded meaning that goes beyond the obvious? What are the ethical implications arising from such a request?

2. On the assumption that Dr. P.K., the attending neonatologist, was unaware of the father's request not to take extraordinary measures to prolong the child's life, did she act in a moral fashion?

3. On the assumption that Dr. P.K. was aware of the father's request, did she act in a moral fashion?

4. Since parents are ethically and legally entitled to make medical decisions for their children and, given that the father in this case is a physician, what moral judgment can be rendered on the action taken by Dr. M.?

5. From an ethical perspective what can be said about the apparent absence of consultation with the baby's mother?

6. From the perspective of interaction with other medical practitioners, how can Dr. M.'s action in dismissing the nurses be categorized?

7. Were the nurses justified in leaving their post?

Reference

Chira, S. 1994. New medical quandary at heart of a trial. *The New York Times*, Aug. 3, p.17.

CASE 9.23
Profits Versus Patient Care

In every business venture there is a constant tension between service and the bottom line. As the level of service increases, which costs more to implement, the amount of profit earned for the company and, where applicable, its shareholders decreases commensurately. What are the consequences and ethical implications of this "truism" when applied to a managed health care situation, such as a health maintenance organization (HMO), where peoples' health and, more drastically, even their lives are at stake?

For more than six years the physicians at Ms. K.S.'s (not her real name) HMO, Family Health Plan Cooperative of Milwaukee (Herbert, 1994, 4.19) kept telling her that she was fine. During that period of time (as Ms. K.S. aged from twenty-two to twenty-eight years), she complained of illness constantly but each visit ended with the same pronouncement—she was fine. Exasperated, she went to an independent physician who diagnosed her illness as advanced cervical cancer. Had a proper diagnosis been made when she first complained of illness, "her chances of survival would have been 95% or better" (Herbert, 1994, 4.19), but now that the cancer had spread to many other parts of her body, the prognosis was very grim. It was doubtful that she would live to see her thirtieth birthday.

Ms. K.S., testifying before a congressional committee investigating health care fraud, stated: "Even though my medical records were fully documented with the classic physical characteristics and symptoms of cervical cancer, no doctor or medical practitioner associated with my HMO or its lab ever made the correct diagnosis" (As cited in Herbert, 1994, 4.19). No physician is infallible. Mistakes in diagnosing and prescribing are made occasionally, but to misjudge a well-documented illness for six years is another matter completely. There appears to be a partial explanation for this particular lapse.

During the lengthy period of the patient's illness, three Pap tests and three biopsies were misread by the CBC Clinilab, the lab that did the work for that HMO. To be more accurate, it should be noted that one Pap test was read correctly but apparently the results were dismissed because the biopsy was misread.

The owner of the lab that handled the tests had been a member of the HMO's Board of Directors. He was strategically placed; "in order to receive the HMO's business he was provided with the competitors' bids in advance" (Herbert, 1994, 4.19). This sort of practice encourages (or is *compels* the more accurate descriptor?) the bidder to offer services at artificially low prices.

Questions to consider for discussion

1. Obtaining contracts at such low prices exerts enormous pressure on the technicians employed by the lab. Indeed, the lab technician who misread Ms. K.S.'s Pap smears "had been reading five times the federally recommended slides and working for four other labs simultaneously" (Herbert, 1994, 4.19). When contracts are won at such low prices, "productivity" and "efficiency" must increase exponentially as otherwise the lab will operate at a loss. Wages are depressed and employees are expected to work at superhuman levels. Can the work be done properly, with the appropriate safeguards for accurate results, by technicians who are under such pressure to produce?

2. From an ethical perspective, who should be charged with the responsibilities of setting standards for patient care, including laboratory testing procedures?

3. Since it is the physician who is ultimately responsible for the treatment of the patient, what role should physicians play in the selection and operation of labs used by HMOs?

4. Is it proper, from an ethical perspective, to allow the owner of the lab that does the work for the HMO to be a member of that Board of Directors?

5. What ethical judgment can be rendered on the action of the HMO in providing the owner of the lab with "the competitors' bids in advance"?

Reference

Herbert, B. 1994. Profits before patients. *The New York Times*, Sept. 11, 4.19.

CASE 9.24
Life or Death for a Baby

Baby R.N. was born six weeks premature, asphyxiated with barely a heartbeat. "His doctors at Sacred Heart Medical Center in Spokane, Washington, revived him after heroic efforts" (Kolata, 1994, A1). As is often the case with such infants, many other medical problems were present, including kidney failure, a bowel obstruction and brain damage. In face of all R.N.'s medical problems, the physicians at the Center concluded that aggressive treatment would only serve to prolong his suffering. Since, in their considered opinion, survival beyond infancy was highly unlikely, they suggested that his life support should be withdrawn.

His parents refused to allow treatment to be terminated. They claimed that the medical and hospital staff at Sacred Heart were prepared to allow him to die due to the costs involved, estimated to be $2,000 per day. That charge was vigorously denied by the physicians, who maintained that, from a medical perspective, the case was hopeless due to the presence of so many problems. To complicate matters further, baby R.N.'s parents are members of a visible minority group, and since they were both unemployed, the whole family was on Medicaid.

Other nearby medical centers within Washington State were approached but refused to accept the case, claiming it was futile (Capron, 1995, p.20). Physicians at Legacy Emanuel Children's Hospital in Portland, Oregon, heard about the case and offered to treat him, predicting that he would survive. The baby was transferred there where he would be kept alive by dialysis until such time as that problem could be overcome with a kidney transplant. According to the physicians at Legacy Emanuel, other babies who were much sicker than R.N. were being treated. Furthermore, in their view, with a kidney transplant R.N. had a 75% chance of survival (Kolata, 1994, A12).

Washington's Medicaid program agreed to pay for baby R.N.'s care in Oregon. Had the decision been otherwise, there were clear indications that Oregon's Medicaid program was prepared to pay the costs.

Questions to consider for discussion

1. When should life support be withdrawn, particularly in a case where an infant is involved?

2. What rights do the parents have? What rights should the parents have?

3. What ethical base can be used in making the decision to withdraw life support?

4. Should there be limits placed on the resources a society is willing to devote to saving a life when the odds of survival appear so unfavorable?

5. In predicting the future quality of life for the child, what relative weight should be given to the willingness of parents to undertake "extraordinary" responsibilities in rearing that child? What, if any, consideration should be given to anticipated future communal costs which may be needed to provide an array of special services that the child will need?

6. What are the ethical implications of one medical center agreeing to continue treatment after other centers have recommended the cessation of treatment?

References

Capron, A.M. 1995. Baby Ryan and virtual futility. *Hasting Center Report* 25(2):20-21.

Kolata, G. 1994. Battle over a baby's future raises hard ethical issues. *The New York Times,* Dec. 27, A1, A12.

CASE 9.25

Consulting as Conflict of Interest

Dr. P.H.S. is a nationally known specialist, a professor at Harvard Medical School and former editor of the official journal of the American College in his specialty. This journal is the logical place for articles to be published on the controversial topic of breast implants. In 1994, Dr. S., charging $300 per hour as a consultant to lawyers who worked for the implant makers, earned $30,000 from four law firms (*The New York Times*, Dec. 13, 1994, B10).

During his tenure as editor, spanning approximately four and one-half years, no article critical of implants was published in the journal. In 1992 and 1993, some doctors who believed implants caused disease submitted at least two articles to the journal; both were rejected but published in other journals. Late in 1993, Dr. S and three colleagues submitted their own article to the journal, which was published. In that article the authors concluded that "there is 'little or no association' between implants and disease" (B10). No mention was made of Dr. S.'s consulting work when the article was submitted.

Many medical journals publish standards stating that authors should disclose conflicts of interest and editors should never pass judgment on work involving areas of personal financial interest (*The New York Times*, Dec. 13, 1994, B10). When confronted with the apparent lapse, Dr. S. denied any conflict of interest, noting that he felt no need to disclose his ties with the implant industry because his views were not biased by that association. He is quoted as saying, "I don't think working with any attorney has influenced my medical judgment, my scientific judgment or my editorial judgment" (B10).

Dates are important in this case. Dr. S earned his money as a consultant in 1994. In January 1993, ethical rules adopted "by the International Committee of Journal Editors lists consulting and expert testimony among 'the most important conflicts of interest' regardless of whether the authors' judgments are affected" (B10). As editor of the official journal of one of the major medical specialties, it seems reasonable to assume that Dr. S. was aware of the rules adopted by the International Committee.

Questions to consider for discussion

1. Is it ethical for the editor of a medical journal to submit his own article to that journal?

2. Was it proper for Dr. S. to retain his position as editor even though he supported only one side of a controversial issue?

3. From an ethical perspective, what is the status of Dr. S.'s insistence that his medical, scientific and editorial judgments were not influenced by his consulting work?

4. Did Dr. S. breach an ethical principle by not disclosing his association with the breast implant industry when he submitted the article he wrote with three colleagues to the journal where he was the editor?

Reference

[No Author]. 1994. Ethics issue over doctor as legal consultant. *The New York Times*, Dec. 13, B10.

CASE 9.26
Should There Be a Limit?

California, it has often been said, is a state like no other and a place where unusual things happen. California is the setting for this case which raises some perplexing and unusual ethical questions that arise from recent technological advances.

Julie G., a single woman aged twenty-eight, was diagnosed with acute lymphoblastic leukemia. As soon as the condition was diagnosed chemotherapy was started at City of Hope Hospital in Los Angeles. Shortly after the inauguration of the treatment, Julie became aware that the regimen would make her sterile. Although she had no boyfriend at that time, she had always wanted to be a mother. Convinced that she would beat the disease, Julie took steps to enable her to overcome sterility and become a mother in the future. Modern technology would make that possible.

In August 1994, Julie's chemotherapy was halted to give her body a thirty-day respite before beginning radiation treatment. During that period, "Julie chose to have fertility treatment" (Craig, 1997, F8). Following the fertility treatment, Julie had her eggs harvested. At the appropriate time Julie's father accompanied her to the University of California cryobank in Los Angeles to select a donor. Twelve embryos were frozen for future use. Unfortunately, Julie's dream of becoming a mother ended with her death on December 28, 1996. Or did it?

In Julie's dying weeks, when she was blind and bedridden, Julie's parents "say she gave her blessing to them finding a host mother for her baby after her death" (Craig, 1997, F8). Her mother consented to Julie's request that she have a direct role in raising Julie's child. Mrs. G. vowed to fulfill that promise.

A few months after Julie's death, her parents, having won legal ownership of their daughter's frozen embryos, advertised for a surrogate mother to bear their daughter's baby. That advertisement created an ethical furor over what was described as an attempt to re-create or duplicate their dead daughter. The parents rejected the criticisms, arguing that they had every right to become the grandparents of their dead daughter's child.

Despite the adverse comments, Julie's parents continued their quest to become grandparents. Two attempts at surrogacy failed, and at the time the article was published, the third, and final, attempt was just underway. Unusual consequences could ensue. "If the pregnancy is successful, it will be the first time a surrogate child has been born after the death of the mother" (Craig, 1997, F8). Phrased somewhat differently, it could be claimed that Julie will have become a mother from beyond the grave. Medical history will have been made.

Questions to consider for discussion

1. Sophisticated technology enables the medical community to fertilize eggs from a variety of donors, under a wide range of circumstances, and freeze the embryos for an indefinite length of time. From an ethical perspective, what limits, if any, should be placed on this procedure?

2. What say should physicians have in establishing these limits?

3. In this particular case, assuming that the last implantation succeeded and resulted in a live birth, what consequences does this scenario have for our notion of the family?

4. If the implantation in the first surrogate had succeeded, what would be the proper treatment for the remaining embryos? Who should make that decision?

5. A number of questions emerge from a somewhat different, but critically important, perspective. Who is the patient in this case? What illness does the patient have which requires medical treatment? If there is no illness, what is the ethical rationale for medical intervention? If there is no illness, what ethical justification is there for using scarce medical resources?

Reference

Craig, O. 1997. The right to be grandparents. *The Ottawa Citizen*, Oct. 12, F8.

CASE 9.27
Patient's Rights Versus Physician's Decisions

In modern times the notion of personal autonomy commands much more attention. This feature, often expressed in terms of the patient's rights, has become increasingly important in the determination of treatment. When patients exercise their autonomy by refusing treatment, those decisions are invariably respected, but such cases are not the only instances where patients, or their surrogates, exercise their autonomy. Cases where further treatment is deemed to be futile by the medical staff but demanded by the patient or surrogate are creating both ethical and legal dilemmas. Confounding the situation is the current aggressive thrust toward cost containment found in all forms of health care, including insurance companies, private and cooperative managed health care organizations and the public sector, where government is the single payer.

On June 7, 1987, Mrs. C.F.G., then seventy-one years old, entered hospital to have surgery for a hip fracture. Mrs. G. had many other medical problems, including diabetes, heart disease, chronic urinary tract infection and Parkinson's. Her medical history listed a mastectomy for breast cancer and a stroke the year before. Mrs. G. was not a stranger to hip surgery—one had been replaced twice and the other one once before. Unfortunately, just before the surgery could begin, "she had a seizure and entered into status epilepticus, a condition of repeated and uncontrollable seizures. When these seizures ended, she had irreversible brain damage and was comatose" (Kolata, 1995, B8).

Ms. J.G., the daughter of the patient and, since the onset of the coma, the surrogate, says she told the physicians at the hospital to do everything in their power to keep her mother alive since that was her mother's wish. On July 5, after Mrs. G.'s physicians consulted with the hospital's optimum care committee, a specially constituted group which mediates issues such as this, authorization was given for a Do Not Resuscitate (DNR) order. When the daughter objected, the order was withdrawn. A month later, a new attending physician came on duty and repeated the request to the committee for a DNR order. Permission was granted, and the order was re-entered on the patient's chart on August 7. Three days later, on August 10, Mrs. G. died. Her daughter maintains that, had she known about the new order, she would have objected again immediately, reiterating her demand that everything possible be done to keep her mother alive.

Ms. J.G. launched a lawsuit against the Massachusetts General Hospital in Boston, charging that they acted against her wishes in treating her mother. At the end of the trial, once the judgment is handed down, certain legal precedents for such cases will have been established (Kolata, 1995, B8) where none were present. These anticipated legal precedents will help direct medical practice, but a number of ethical issues will still need to be addressed by medical practitioners involved in such cases.

Within the present climate of cost constraints, doctors' expenditures are being monitored very closely, particularly in managed health care organizations. Physicians who provide futile treatment are held accountable by management for spending too much on their patients and may even incur the risk of dismissal. On the other hand, withholding treatment opens up the risk of a lawsuit. In such cases physicians are placed in an untenable position.

Questions to consider for discussion

1. Were the physicians acting morally when they requested a DNR order from the optimum care committee?

2. Who should determine when further treatment is futile?

3. Is this an appropriate question in light of present technological advances where, with the use of respirators, patients can be kept "alive" indefinitely?

4. Is it fair for family members to insist that patients deemed to be futile cases be kept alive in face of the difficulties a health care team has when working for no possible positive end?

5. Costs for keeping a patient such as Mrs. G. in an intensive care unit run approximately $17,500 per week. Would that be a factor to consider in this case? Should costs for treatment ever be a factor in treating patients?

Reference

Kolata, G. 1995. Withholding care from patients: Boston case asks, who decides? *The New York Times*, April 3, p.1, B8.

CASE 9.28

Public Good or Corporate Profit?

CellPro Inc. is a small Seattle biotechnology company that has created a product which "uses a unique technology to remove cancerous cells and to specifically select healthy, immune-building cells from bone marrow extracted from a patient. The marrow is re-implanted following radiation and chemotherapy" (M. Meyer and T. Weingarten, A deadly serious fight. *Newsweek*, May 19, 1997, p.60). Trial tests carried out on five thousand patients over two years have proven effective in treating diseases such as multiple sclerosis and various forms of cancer. Clinical trials to treat other diseases using the new technology are underway at scores of medical centers across the United States and in Europe.

In 1996, CellPro's president was diagnosed as having a rare type of lymphoma and was given less than two years to live. He became CellPro's first human test case, and, a year later, appeared to be cancer-free. CellPro's innovation has been hailed as "one of the biggest breakthroughs in transplant therapy in the last decade" (Meyer and Weingarten, 1997, p.60) by a medical researcher at Emory University. Its potential as a treatment for a number of diseases appears to be very promising and will become a reality only if certain legal impediments can be overcome.

Baxter International, a giant pharmaceutical company, has sued CellPro for an infringement on one of its patents. Baxter insists that CellPro remove its therapy from the market or, if it continues to offer the treatment, that all the profits should revert to them. Removing the therapy from the market would leave thousands of patients, and many more potential patients, abandoned, because CellPro is the only one that makes the product. Baxter is at least one year away from receiving regulatory approval for its own technology (Meyer & Weingarten, 1997, p.60). Handing over the profits earned on the treatment to Baxter would bankrupt CellPro, putting it out of business and leaving a clear path for Baxter to capture the entire market.

Large sums of money are involved. One biotech analyst estimates that if the technology passes all the required tests it could become a $100 million dollar business in a very short time.

A trial in the spring of 1997 failed to settle matters. The jury in the case found in favor of CellPro but was overruled by the judge who held "that CellPro had knowingly used technology patented by John Hopkins University and licenced by Baxter" (Meyer and Weingarten, 1997, p.60). Siding with the jury are many medical researchers. Given the results of the trial, the president of CellPro, a beneficiary of his company's therapy, expressed confidence that they would prevail on appeal.

Because this therapy appears to be so promising, political intervention was sought to ensure that the product remains available. Four U.S. senators, along with the president of the American Cancer Society, petitioned the Secretary of the Department of Health and Human Services to compel Baxter to extend a licence to CellPro in the public interest.

Questions to consider for discussion

1. From an ethical perspective, what judgment should be rendered on CellPro if, in fact, it did infringe on one of Baxter's patents?

2. If CellPro did, in fact, infringe on one of Baxter's patents, is the demand that CellPro either stop distributing the technology or, if it continues, hand over the profits, fair?

3. What ethical judgment can be rendered on Baxter's action in suing CellPro if, in fact, there was no patent infringement?

4. On the assumption that CellPro did infringe on one of Baxter's patents, but taking into account the public good, what would be a fair solution for all the parties involved?

Reference

Meyer, M., and T. Weinstein. 1997. A deadly serious fight. *Newsweek*, May 19, p.60.

CASE 9.29

Humanitarian Intervention or Opportunity Missed?

Death, as a concept, was reconceptualized in 1968 with the publication of the report prepared by the Harvard Medical School, which recommended whole brain death as the defining criterion. Many, but not all, in the medical community have come to accept this standard. However, within the public realm the situation is much different. In this realm there is a much greater reluctance to accept brain death as the standard, particularly in cases where the patient is attached to a ventilator and appears to be breathing, a sign associated with life.

Establishing valid and acceptable criteria for the determination of death has both legal and ethical implications. In political jurisdictions where the law is not crystal clear—and even where the law appears to be clear—cases tried by the court establish precedents which help define acceptable practices. Delays, such as the one described in the forthcoming case, may only serve to postpone badly needed decisions, even if the motivation to help a family is based on good intentions.

Infant M.S., aged five months and very ill, was admitted to Long Island Jewish Medical Center where she was attached to a ventilator. A short time thereafter, physicians at the Center, using brain death as the criterion, pronounced the baby dead. A week later, lawyers went to court seeking authorization to cease treatment for a patient who was legally a corpse. The parents objected. Publicity given to the case prompted John Cardinal O'Connor, the Roman Catholic Archbishop of New York, to intercede by arranging for the infant to be transferred to a Roman Catholic hospital, St.Vincent's, in Manhattan. There she would be attached to a ventilator and kept alive.

In effecting the transfer to St. Vincent's, the Cardinal indicated that the Church was ready to bear the costs if the parents' insurance company refused to pay for the infant's hospital care. Although unstated, it was presumed that the infant would stay on the ventilator "until such time as her heart stopped beating" (Bruni, 1994, B2).

Experts testified that it was impossible to estimate how long the heart of a brain-dead baby attached to a ventilator could continue beating. In one documented case "a brain dead baby on a ventilator showed vital signs for 5 years, 3 months" (Bruni, 1996, B2). Further comments were added: In certain cases a brain-dead child's body underwent serious decomposition before the heart finally ceased beating. Keeping a brain-dead baby in the intensive care unit was regarded as a macabre injustice for physicians, nurses and the families of the other infants there; they were compelled to endure the presence of a legally dead baby in their midst.

Transferring the infant put an end to the opportunity to hear legal arguments which would "clarify a fuzzy phrase in state regulations that requires hospitals to make 'reasonable accommodation' for families who on religious grounds do not accept the medical and legal principle that brain death constitutes death" (Bruni, 1996, B1).

Some Orthodox Jewish leaders and American Indians have formally objected to equating brain death with death. In the United States, Roman Catholic officials have not taken such a position. A much stronger stand was taken in Germany, where a statement published early in 1994 by the bishops of the Evangelical (Protestant) church rejected that criterion. "They considered brain death to be an invention of transplant surgeons for their own purposes, and that by itself was not real death" (Nicholson, 1994, p.5). In April of the same year, the Roman Catholic bishops of Germany adopted the same view. Simply obeying the law does not necessarily avert the ethical issue involved.

Clarification of the wording of any statute or regulation is obviously important, because those rulings serve as guidelines for proper behavior. Even after the wording is clarified, difficult ethical issues may still need to be addressed.

Questions to consider for discussion

1. Were the lawyers for the Long Island Jewish Medical Center right to petition the court?

2. From an ethical perspective, was Cardinal O'Connor's intervention justified? Was it the right thing to do?

3. Did the transfer of the infant to St. Vincent's really help anyone?

4. By agreeing to admit the infant, who was pronounced dead, did St. Vincent's behave in an ethical manner?

5. Can the costs involved and the use of scarce medical resources be justified?

6. What would you do if, as a medical practitioner who does not accept brain death as the equivalence of death, you were asked by the family of your patient to remove him or her from life support after brain death has been ascertained?

References

Bruni, F. 1996. Baby's move ends a battle over her fate. *The New York Times,* Mar. 1, B1, B2.

Nicholson, R.H. 1994. The good received, the giver is forgot. *Hastings Center Report* 24(4):5.

CASE 9.30
Whose Needs Come First?

A local pediatrician, employed by a national HMO,[1] referred a three-month-old girl to the pediatric-oncology group at the University of North Carolina Hospitals in Chapel Hill. She was found to have leucocytosis, anemia and thrombocytopenia, resulting in a diagnosis of acute lymphoblastic leukemia (Weston and Lauria, 1996, p.543). Intensive chemotherapy was started immediately. A bone marrow transplant, with the older sister as donor, was recommended in the first remission. Even with transplantation treatment, the prognosis for such patients is guarded.

The HMO approved the recommended treatment. They requested the University Hospitals' assistance in transferring the baby to the nearest "center of quality" (Weston and Lauria, 1996, p.543), a transplantation center located in another state. Despite there being two excellent transplantation centers in North Carolina, much closer to Chapel Hill, this center had been selected by the HMO to perform all bone marrow transplantations in the region. When that decision was reported to the parents by the attending oncologist and the social worker, the enormous difficulties facing the family became clear. Due to employment commitments, the father would not be able to accompany his family, and the mother, who obviously needed to be with her infant, would lose her position and upon her return be forced to take a lesser job with a lower rate of pay. To further aggravate matters, the older sister was having serious behavioral problems. A prolonged absence from the mother would surely exacerbate an already problematic situation. With neither family nor friends in the out-of-state city, the expenses involved in a prolonged stay would be difficult for the family to manage.

In response to a request, the medical team at UNC Hospitals asked the HMO to make an exception in this case. The HMO refused. This response prompted further investigation by the attending

---

[1] In the op-ed article by Bob Herbert in *The New York Times*, he points out that the HMO was not identified in the Weston and Lauria article and, at their request, the name is being withheld in his own piece. He notes that HMOs have been known to retaliate against critics.

oncologist into the rationale provided by the HMO; namely, that it examines the results of transplantations at all centers and selects only the "best" for its clients. During the probe it was found that Johns Hopkins University and the University of Minnesota were not among this select group. "It turned out that the center selected for our patient has no particular expertise in acute lymphoblastic leukemia in infants or in the preparative regimen or transplantation procedure" (Weston and Lauria, 1996, p.543). Members of the University Hospitals team could not find any published reports from the Center chosen by the HMO to indicate medical reasons for its selection.

Colleagues at the University Hospitals cautioned against pushing the HMO too far since that action might jeopardize their chances of being selected as a center in the future. Instead of complaining, the HMO told them they "should be glad we cover this procedure. Get used to it. Its happening everywhere. Your program may end up being a beneficiary of this approach" (Weston and Lauria, 1996, p.543). None of the HMO's responses addressed the specific needs of the patient and her family. Furthermore, the HMO complained about the University Hospitals' interference with the client-carrier relationship (Herbert, 1996, A29).

With no alternative available, the family complied with the arrangements made by the HMO. The baby and mother went to the out-of-state center where the transplantation was carried out successfully. Six months passed before the baby was returned into the care of her physicians in North Carolina. During that period, the sister lived with relatives in another state. As anticipated, the mother was demoted and, to make an already difficult situation worse, the father lost his job.

Several weeks later, the baby suffered a relapse. Chemotherapy was re-introduced and a second bone marrow transplantation contemplated. The "HMO, for reasons having nothing to do with the quality of care, recommended a different transplant center in yet another state" (Herbert, 1996, A29). This decision disregarded the family's psychosocial and economic straits and the previously established relationship between the patient and the first transplantation center. As well, the infant's primary oncologist and social worker were effectively removed from the decision-making loop.

Due to this ordeal, the parents have lost their home and their savings, and the older sister has had increasingly severe behavioral problems. When faced with a second extended stay in another state, in order to keep the family together, the mother quit her job, gave up her HMO coverage and applied for Medicaid.

Questions to consider for discussion

1. What ethical judgment can be rendered on the decisions made by the HMO to refer the infant patient to out-of-state transplantation centers?

2. What ethical judgment can be rendered on the HMO in referring the infant to a different center for the second transplantation?

3. Were Dr. Weston and Ms. Lauria right in attempting to have the infant referred to an in-state center?

4. Is it proper for a university-hospital based physician to interfere in the client-carrier relationship?

5. What ethical judgment can be rendered on Dr. Weston's colleagues, who cautioned him against offending the carrier "because we are in the running for the next contract"?

6. Was the mother right in quitting her job, giving up her HMO coverage and applying for Medicaid?

References

Herbert, B. 1996. Torture by H.M.O. *The New York Times*, Mar. 15, A29.

Weston, B., and M. Lauria. 1996. Patient advocacy in the 1990s. *New England Journal of Medicine* 334(8):543-544.

CASE 9.31
Royalties Versus the Public Good

There was a time when what mattered most to medical researchers was altruism and pride in discovering something that would benefit humankind. When a substance was developed or a new link discovered, the researchers rushed to publish their findings in medical journals in order to alert the scientific world. At present it appears that we are living in a new era, with a new ethos, where royalties sometimes take precedence over the public good.

Dr. M.B. was working in a lab at the University of California at San Diego in 1986 when he noticed a relationship in the test results of pregnant women between the levels of a frequently checked hormone, human chorionic gonadotropin, or HCG, and Down syndrome. After the university declined to patent the "discovery," Dr. B. filed with the office himself. Some time passed, and the patent was granted in 1989. During the interim, in 1987, Dr. B. published a paper describing his findings.

At that time, Dr. B.'s finding was of limited value in and of itself, because the test produced too many false positives. This factor made the test unacceptable as a diagnostic tool. Very soon thereafter, in 1988, "a team of researchers reported that a test for three natural substances in pregnancy, including HCG, was far more useful in detecting true cases of Down syndrome without high number of false positives" (Eichenwald, 1997, D3). The other markers are Alpha fetoprotein (ATP) and Estriol, with the age of the mother serving as an important factor. With the reduction of the previously high false positives, the triple blood screen rapidly became commonplace in the early weeks of pregnancy. Positive results from this test prompts physicians to recommend that their patients undergo amniocentesis, a more expensive and invasive procedure, to confirm the diagnosis.

Shortly after Dr. B received his patent in 1989, he approached labs conducting the triple blood screen and demanded royalty payments for those screens which include the HCG test. Since the HCG test had been used for decades, for other purposes as well, his demands were ignored. Dr. B. was not to be denied; various avenues were explored to enable him to exact royalties.

In the fall of 1996, lawyers for Dr. B.'s company contacted the Foundation for Blood Research, a non-profit Maine laboratory that is one of the largest in the United States. A proposition was offered: a percentage of the royalties would be given to the lab "if it disclosed which labs around the country participated in a quality assurance program it conducts for the screening" (Eichenwald, 1997, D3). At first the Foundation rejected the offer outright. A lawyer for the Foundation wrote, "Your proposal is in direct conflict with the interests and rights of patients and physicians and the public at large" (Eichenwald, 1997, D3). However, when threatened with a patent infringement suit, they did an about-face and accepted the offer. Citing "a business decision" as the rationale, a licensing agreement was signed. With a list of labs using the test and one signed licensing agreement in hand, Dr. B.'s lawyers were in a much stronger position to go after other labs.

Groups facing a patent infringement suit often choose to settle, even if they believe the patent or the charge to be invalid. Since all patents have the presumption of validity in the eyes of the court, a defendant must prove the contrary, an endeavor which could become exceedingly expensive. If the defendant loses, additional dire consequences may ensue—the patent holder can petition for an injunction to prevent future infringements. In this case, if an injunction were to be obtained, it could effectively shut down blood screenings until the labs agreed to royalty terms.

The legal costs involved in fighting a patent infringement suit and the potentially steep down side if the ruling goes against the defendant have a tendency to terrorize those accused of infringement. From a strictly financial or business perspective, it may be more prudent to settle matters even if there is great doubt about the validity of the accusation of infringement.

Some legal experts predicted that a court would probably invalidate the patent, since "Dr. Bogart did not, in fact, invent anything in the traditional sense. Rather, he was granted his patent as a result of his noticing a natural function in the body that likely has existed since the dawn of man" (Eichenwald, 1997, D3). Despite the doubts, and despite the fact that a dangerous precedent was about to be set, it appears that the financial costs involved in fighting a law suit served as a major deterrent.

Late in June 1997, letters from Dr. B.'s attorney, who is working on contingency, began arriving in labs across the United States. They were given less than two weeks to agree to licensing agreements. Those who agreed were granted a benefit, a release from liability for royalties owed in the past. Those who refused to comply would be sued for the full amount.

Under a complex formula devised by Dr. B. and his attorney, labs could pay anywhere from $5 to $9 per test. Reimbursement from Medicaid and private insurers would not cover the added costs, thus placing the labs in an untenable position. They could either seek higher payments, which most likely would not be forthcoming, or they could stop doing the tests. Yet without these tests the health of countless pregnant women would be put at risk.

Condemnation of Dr. B.'s actions have been voiced by highly respected members of the medical community, who have pointed out the adverse effects on public health. In rebuttal "Dr. Bogart said that the labs were simply attempting to profit from his patent without paying the money they legally owe him" (Eichenwald, 1997, D3). It was obviously unfair for these labs to be making large profits while the one who provided the test is being denied the opportunity to earn money from his patent. There is no coercion involved, since the labs are not forced to continue doing the screening.

Large sums of money are involved. A.D., the lawyer representing Dr. B.'s company, commented that his client stood to earn as much as $100 million during the life of the patent. Although the amount of money seems large, it is merited because of the potential benefit to millions and millions of pregnant women.

Questions to consider for discussion

1. Did the University of California at San Diego act properly in refusing to file for the patent?

2. Did Dr. B. act ethically in obtaining this patent?

3. Did Dr. B. behave ethically in threatening to sue all the labs if they did not sign licensing agreements with his company?

4. Did the Foundation for Blood Research behave properly?

5. Did they really have an alternative?

References

Marshall, E. 1990. When commerce and academe collide. *Science* 248(4952):152-156.

Witt, M.D., and L.O. Gosten. 1994. Conflict of interest dilemmas in biomedical research. *Journal of the American Medical Association* 271(7):547-551.

Eichenwald, E. 1997. Push for royalties threatens use of down syndrome test. *The New York Times*, May 23, p.1, D3.

CASE 9.32

Palliation, Quality of Life, Costs Involved

A previously active sixty-one-year-old gentleman, A.T., had recently been confined to a wheelchair by progressive osteoarthritis in his right hip. Along with the pain came considerable distress at his lack of mobility and loss of independence. A hip replacement would relieve his pain, increase his mobility and significantly improve his quality of life. His insurance company had agreed to pay the costs. In light of the anticipated benefits, he decided to proceed with elective surgery.

Except for the osteoarthritis, A.T. considered himself to be in excellent health. He attributed his recent decrease in stamina to his joint disease. A preoperative blood count suggested that he had chronic lymphocytic leukemia (CLL) and associated moderate anemia. "A thorough work up confirmed the diagnosis of Stage III CLL, which is associated with a life expectancy of approximately twelve to forty-two months" (*Hastings Center Report*, 1992, p.41). Periodic blood transfusions, in the opinion of his physicians, would correct the anemia.

Although his newly diagnosed condition posed no threat to the success of his hip replacement surgery, the hospital and the insurance company questioned the cost of a hip replacement for a patient who was now in palliative care.

Questions to consider for discussion

1. What ethical rationale can be provided for proceeding with the hip replacement surgery?

2. What ethical rationale can be provided for canceling the hip replacement surgery?

3. What role does (or should) the patient play in this decision?

4. What role does (or should) the physician play in this decision?

5. What role does (or should) the hospital play in this decision?

6. What role does (or should) the insurance company play in this decision?

7. What, if any, are the ethical implications of categorizing this, or any, patient as being in palliative care?

8. What are the limits of palliation in the age of chronic disease?

9. How can the greatest good for the greatest number be served in this case? Can more than one utilitarian alternative be argued?

10. How does Kant's categorical imperative apply in this case?

References

[No Author]. 1992. Palliation in the age of chronic disease. *Hastings Center Report* 22(1):41.

Fins, J.J. 1992. Commentary. *Hastings Center Report* 22(1):41-42.

Callahan, D. 1992. Commentary. *Hastings Center Report* 22(1):42.

CASE 9.33

Cultural Relativism and Western Medical Practice

How far should Western medical practitioners go in attempting to understand other cultures and, perhaps more important, what degree of tolerance should be used in accepting certain healing practices that differ from our approach?

Ms. S., an immigrant from Laos who had been in the United States for more than a decade, brought her youngest child into the clinic for her four-month immunizations. Marie is a lively, healthy infant, who is progressing normally. Dr. Leigh, the attending physician, had learned much about the Iu Mien culture of Ms. S.'s native Laos from a number of their previous conversations. This knowledge has enabled Dr. Leigh to better understand the many Mien patients living in the vicinity who visit the clinic for some of their medical needs.

Ms. S. experienced some turbulent times when she first came to United States but now, as a married woman, she seemed well adjusted. At this point in her life she took pride in being a Mien woman (*Hastings Center Report*, 1993, p.15) and her growing knowledge of Mien traditions and beliefs. She was happy to share her knowledge of Mien spirits, ceremonies and cures with Dr. Leigh during visits to the clinic. In this visit, Ms. S. did not hesitate to explain the meaning of the burns on her baby's stomach.

Dr. Leigh was somewhat incredulous as she looked at the five red and blistered quarter-inch round markings on the baby's abdomen. Ms. S. explained that this was a traditional cure for a case of "Gusia mun toe," a rare folk illness among Mien babies, characterized by restlessness, continual crying, agitation, constipation and loss of appetite. Throwing the head back when held is a tell-tale characteristic of the syndrome.

How the cure is administered was explained. The "string" of the inner pulp found in a special reed is dipped lightly into pork fat and then lit. As the flame is passed quickly over the skin above the pain site, some of the hot fat drops and raises a blister that pops, like popcorn, indicating that the illness is not related to spiritual causes. If no blisters arise, the services of a shaman may be needed to conduct a spiritual ritual to effect a cure. Other components of this traditional cure include the symbolic transfer of pain to an inanimate object such as a wall.

Ms. S. explained that the original pain usually subsides within a half-hour and any pain from the burns is gone within an hour. Infection is rare, and the scars generally disappear in a week or so. She acknowledged that this method of cure was dangerous for children. Dr. Leigh concurred with the assessment but soon discovered that their understanding of danger in this instance differed considerably due to cultural differences. Ms. S. tried to allay Dr. Leigh's concerns by explaining that the cure was done by her mother-in-law, who was highly skilled in the procedure. Best of all, the baby had stopped crying immediately after the procedure, calmed down and regained her appetite.

Dr. Leigh proceeded with her examination of the baby and found no reason to question the mother's assessment. As Dr. Leigh administered the infant's immunizations, she became acutely aware "that the procedure considerably disturbed the baby's contentment, and wondering—not for the first time—about the pain she routinely inflicted upon children in the course of her practice" (*Hastings Center Report*, 1993, p.15). Dr. Leigh had not voiced her misgivings about Ms. S.'s practice of inflicting burns on her baby. As the visit ended, she wondered if she had done the right thing by remaining silent.

Questions to consider for discussion

1. On the assumption that the local jurisdiction has a law requiring all professionals, physicians included, to report suspected instances of child abuse, did Dr. Leigh behave properly in not reporting the incident to the authorities?

2. Was Dr. Leigh right in not voicing her misgivings? Should she have said something even if it meant intruding on a different culture?

3. In a medical setting, to what extent can other cultural practices be accommodated?

References

1993. Culture, healing, and professional obligations. *Hastings Center Report* 23(4):15.

Carrese, J. 1993. Commentary. *Hastings Center Report* 23(4):16.

Brown, K., and A. Jameton. 1993. Commentary. *Hastings Center Report* 23(4):17.

Ehrenreich, J.D. 1996. Worms, witchcraft and wild incantations: The case of the chicken soup cure. *Anthropological Quarterly* 69(3):137-141.

CASE 9.34

Professional Courtesy, Professional Impropriety and Authenticity

To raise one's voice or to remain silent in the face of another physician's misconduct or impropriety is one of the most difficult ethical dilemmas a clinician will face. This predicament is difficult enough when the practitioners involved are of the same professional status. The quandary is exacerbated in situations where the alleged impropriety is committed by a senior clinician, and the one questioning the behavior is a junior who is dependent on the senior clinician's evaluation and recommendation for career advancement. Speaking up infringes upon the implicit agreement not to embarrass or impugn the reputation of a colleague. Speaking up also carries great personal risks. Remaining silent causes problems for the individual and for the profession as a whole. Where such incidents occur in a medical setting, it is invariably the patient, and members of the family, who suffer.

Medicine has undergone dramatic scientific and technological changes in the past half-century. Changes in thinking have also transformed the physician-patient relationship. Paternalism, physician knows what is best for you (Charon et al., 1996, p.252), has been replaced by a more egalitarian approach. Students today are taught about patient autonomy and empowerment. Emphasis is placed on involving the patient in making decisions based upon information provided by the medical team. In actual practice a "generation gap" may exist as physicians from "the old school" conduct themselves in ways that are different from what is being taught currently in medical schools. It appears that a fresh medical clerk found himself in a situation involving all of the factors noted above.

Abdominal pain of four days duration prompted a thirty-four-year-old patient to visit her obstetrician/gynecologist. Since her last menstrual period had been twenty-six days before, she suspected she was pregnant. Her urine pregnancy test was positive, and a trans-vaginal ultrasound indicated a mass in the right fallopian tube. The ultrasound result confirmed the finding in the physical examination. Her past surgical history was significant for two ectopic pregnancies and a left salpingectomy.

The obstetrician/gynecologist advised the patient that he sus-pected an ectopic pregnancy and discussed the possible risks and consequences with the patient. "He suggested that since she al-ready had one child she should consider having a tubal ligation to preclude harm to herself" (Jones, 1996, p.753). After listening care-fully, the patient consented to the removal of the ectopic pregnancy but deferred a decision on the tubal ligation until she had discussed matters with her husband. Laparoscopic surgery was scheduled for the next morning.

Prior to surgery the patient and her husband met with the obste-trician/gynecologist, a third-year resident and a first-year clerk. The patient and her husband had considered the matter very carefully and "were resolute in their desire to have another child and did not want the tubal ligation" (Jones, 1996, p.753). In reply to their appeal that everything be done to save the remaining tube, the obstetri-cian/gynecologist said he would do his best. The medical team left and, once out of earshot of the patient, the obstetrician/gynecologist "remarked that they were making the wrong decision, that they would be better off adopting another child, and that he was 'almost certain' that he would be unable to save the tube" (Jones, 1996, p.753).

We are given a report of what transpired during the operation by the clinical clerk:

> Gross visualization of the anatomical structures revealed an absent left fal-lopian tube, normal uterus, and right fallopian tube with a spherical 2 cm intraliminal mass distending the ampullary portion of the tube. Based on observation alone, Dr. Smith declared the tube unsalvageable and proceeded to perform a salpingectomy. Biopsy of the mass in the operating room, however, showed that the tissue was not consistent with an ectopic preg-nancy. The question thus remained: where was the fertilized egg indicated by the positive laboratory tests? A second look at the entire anatomical field revealed no indications of ectopic growth; the pregnancy, I reasoned, must be intrauterine and the ultrasound did not detect it. Dr. Smith ordered the resident to perform a dilation and evacuation (D&E) of the conceptus.

> I was confused. I turned to Dr. Smith and asked him with the candor of a first-year clerk: "Knowing that this is not an ectopic and most probably an intrauterine pregnancy, and knowing that the patient and her husband desire

to have another child, what are the indications for a D&E?" Taken aback by such a blunt question, Dr. Smith paused, and turned a baleful look upon me. No words were spoken, but my most worrisome suspicions were seemingly confirmed. He could have merely removed the contents of the tube, but he didn't. He could have left the D&E for another day following discussion of the unforeseen findings with the patient and her husband, but he didn't. Chorionic villi were observed in the excised uterine lining (Jones, 1996, p.753).

To help extricate himself from this ethical dilemma, the clinical clerk sought counsel from his superiors. He first approached the resident who had assisted in the operation. Although the resident was also troubled by the events during surgery that morning, he was unwilling to take action. Two members of the faculty were approached; the scenario was presented to them as a hypothetical situation to ensure anonymity. There would be no professional embarrassment nor would any reputation be impugned. "Both, without supporting the hypothetical MD, minimized the ethical considerations and attempted to provide clinical indications that might explain Dr. Smith's[1] actions" (Jones, 1996, p.754). Those evasive replies left the clinical clerk with the impression that medical ethics is best confined to the university lecture hall.

As he pondered the situation, the clinical clerk felt alone, isolated, and defeated in his quest for justice. He decided not to bring the situation to light, not to fight the system by himself. Lawsuits would surely ensue as a result of his accusations. Given his lowly professional status and the refusal of others to get involved, he realized that standing alone he could not win.

Questions to consider for discussion

1. Was the obstetrician/gynecologist justified in performing a salpingectomy?

2. From an ethical perspective, what alternatives did he have?

3. Was the clinical clerk right in challenging the obstetrician/gynecologist during the surgery?

4. Was the clinical clerk right in seeking counsel from the third-year resident?

---

[1] The names of the individuals involved have been changed.

5. Was the resident right in refusing to take action?

6. Was the clinical clerk right in deciding not to raise the matter publicly?

7. Was he justified in reasoning that his lowly status made it impossible for him to win a legal battle that would surely result from his exposé?

8. From an existential perspective, did the obstetrician/gynecologist behave in an authentic way?

9. Did the third-year resident?

10. Did the clinical clerk?

References

Jones, T.R. 1996. Speak no evil: Physician silence in the face of professional impropriety. *Journal of the American Medical Association* 276(9):753-754.

Charon, R., H. Brody, M.W. Clark, D. Davis, R. Martinez, and R.M. Nelson. 1996. Literature and ethical medicine: Five cases from common practice. *Journal of Medicine and Philosophy* 21(3):243-265.

CASE 9.35
Profitable Medicine

Certain diseases require specialists' attention based on their lengthy experience in treating that malady. At times, first-class treatment for such illnesses requires a team of specialists familiar with the disease, who are capable of cooperating in a multidisciplinary setting. Two such diseases are sickle-cell anemia, which occurs most often in black people, and thalassemia, which is frequently found in people of Mediterranean and Southeast Asian origin. Both are genetic blood disorders. Since a large proportion of this population resides in the urban centers of the United States, it is usually the physicians who work in inner-city clinics or hospitals who have the most experience in treating these illnesses.

Sickle-cell anemia is a complex disease that affects most of the organs of the body. Patients are vulnerable to heart attacks, liver damage, strokes and other problems. In Oakland, California, Dr. E.V. runs a large program at Children's Hospital devoted to treating sickle-cell anemia and thalassaemia. He was treating a teen-age girl with sickle-cell anemia, whose mother was on welfare. Dr. E.V. "noted that some sickle-cell patients suffer from hemiplegia, a paralysis affecting one side of the body that is caused by a blockage of blood vessels in the brain" (Herbert, 1996, A13). His experience led him to conclude that in such cases aggressive treatment—frequent blood transfusions with normal blood—prevents the events mentioned above from happening.

His teen-aged patient was given frequent transfusions and responded well. Her mother got a job, went off welfare and, through her employment, enrolled in a health maintenance organization (HMO). At this point her daughter was assigned to the care of a hematologist in a suburban hospital, where neither the physician nor the hospital had much experience in treating sickle-cell patients. "The new doctor decided that there was not enough evidence that the frequent transfusions were necessary. He stopped them" (Herbert, 1996, A13). Alarmed, the mother contacted Dr. E.V. for help. He presented a summary of the scientific evidence in support of frequent transfusions to the hematologist and the HMO. They were unmoved.

Another physician's assistance was enlisted. He supported Dr. V.'s recommendation. The HMO and its physician would not relent. Unfortunately this story ends tragically—the girl suffered a stroke and died. Commenting on this event, and other horror stories associated with managed care, Bob Herbert (1996, A13) asks, "Who doubted for even the merest moment that financial incentives to deny medical treatment would result in the widespread denial of medical treatment?" A physician cannot have the patient's best interest at heart knowing that a referral to a specialist or hospitalizing the patient will cost the physician money. This obvious conflict destroys the physician-patient relationship.

Reports of cases such as the one described above have fomented a strong reaction in some parts of the United States. "In the first large organized backlash against what they call the industrialization of medicine, many doctors of Massachusetts' renowned medical schools and teaching hospitals are calling for a moratorium on takeovers of health services and for curbs on the companies' intrusion into doctors' decision-making" (Kilborn, 1997, A12). An organization has emerged, the Ad Hoc Committee to Defend Health Care, chaired by Dr. Bernard Lown, a cardiologist and Harvard professor who shared a Nobel Peace Prize for organizing physicians against nuclear war.

By the middle of June 1997, "1,940 Massachusetts doctors, young and old, men and women, liberal and conservative, most with ties to Harvard, had signed the committee's 'Call to Action'" (Kilborn, 1997, A12).

Other protest actions have been reported. In California and Florida, a few thousand physicians have joined unions to challenge the power of the managed health care corporations.

Dr. Lown's group acknowledges that business efficiency is essential in health care these days "but not to the extent that it compromises the doctor's oath to put the patient first" (Kilborn, 1997, A12). With the onset of managed care, physicians' "productivity" began to be measured. Quotas were set. Physicians surpassing their goals would receive bonuses, but if targets were not met, their pay would be reduced. In many situations, primary care physicians are penalized financially if they make referrals to specialists or hospitalize their patients.

Other aspects are also troublesome. One physician, a member of the Ad Hoc Committee, who has surpassed his goal by the highest proportion of any doctor in his group, highlights the increase in the amount of paperwork required and the bureaucratic second-guessing. "'It seemed more pragmatic', Dr. Stoeckle said. 'But it's always cost, cost, cost'" (Kilborn, 1997, A13). In the drive to reduce costs, lesser-paid nurse-practitioners and physicians' assistants provide more care, and patients are sent out of town for tests where fees are lower. Even the medications prescribed by physicians are second-guessed.

A rebuttal against the Ad Hoc Committee and its Call to Action was voiced by Robert Hughes, president of the Massachusetts Association of HMOs. He claimed that the protest was concentrated among liberal doctors with a political agenda, who were age-old critics of the medical establishment. "Their anger over profit-making is misplaced, Mr. Hughes said, because any health care service, even a doctor's private practice, must receive more in revenue than it spends to stay in business" (Kilborn, 1997, A12). He added that even a church has to make a profit.

Questions to consider for discussion

1. Is it ethical to earn profits from the illness of others?

2. Is it ethical for HMOs to structure contracts with physicians that provide incentives for seeing more patients and penalties for referrals to specialists and hospitalizing patients?

3. Are all for-profit corporate health management organizations in a permanent conflict-of-interest position?

4. Is it ethical for physicians to join unions?

References

Herbert, B. 1996. Hidden agenda. *The New York Times,* July 15, A13.

Kilborn, P.T. 1997. Doctors organize to fight corporate intrusion. *The New York Times,* July 1, A12.

CASE 9.36
Medically Expensive Religious Belief

Enshrined in the First Amendment to the U.S. Constitution is respect for the free exercise of all religious beliefs (Post, 1995, p.28). To what extent should such beliefs be respected when heavy financial demands are placed on medical facilities?

Immediate surgery was recommended to a young woman in her twenties, a Jehovah's Witness, who was diagnosed with an ectopic pregnancy. Prior to the surgery, she was advised that there was a good chance she would need to be transfused. "She unequivocally refused transmission in accord with her religious faith, even after being told that such refusal might result in her death (*Hastings Center Report*, 1995, p.28). As anticipated, she experienced very serious blood loss, with her hemoglobin dropping to three. She was very near death.

Immediate action was required to save her life. A radical procedure was attempted which involved deliberately putting her into a chemical coma, thus paralyzing her and slowing down her life processes. She was placed on a ventilator in the ICU where she stayed for two weeks. She was given a very expensive drug, Neupogen, to address the hemoglobin problem. Her life was saved, at a cost approaching $100,000, which had to be absorbed by the hospital. Spending $100,000 to meet the need of one patient meant that the hospital had that much less available to look after other uninsured individuals who needed medical attention (Fleck, 1995, p.29).

Questions to consider for discussion

1. Was it right for the hospital to spend $100,000 on one patient due to his or her religious beliefs, when standard procedures involved an expenditure of a small fraction of that sum?

2. Is it fair to other uninsured patients?

3. From an ethical perspective, is there a limit to the amount of money that ought to be spent for special treatment on a patient due to religious belief?

References

[No Author]. My conscience, your money. *Hastings Center Report* 25(5):28.

Post, S.G. 1995. Commentary. *Hastings Center Report* 25(5):28.

Fleck, L. 1995. Commentary. *Hastings Center Report* 25(5):29.

Kluge, E.W. 1992. *Biomedical Ethics: In a Canadian Context.* Scarborough, Ont.: Prentice-Hall, Inc.

References

Angell, M. 1991. The case of Helga Wangle: A new kind of "right to die" case. *New England Journal of Medicine* 325:511-512.

Aristotle. 1968. *The Basic Works of Aristotle* (R. McKeon, trans.). New York: Random House

Associated Press. 1995. MDs urge probe of baboon marrow transplant. *The Globe and Mail*. December 19, A13.

Bard, T.R. 1990. *Medical Ethics in Practice*. New York: Hemisphere Publishing Corporation.

Barry, V. 1982. *Moral Aspects of Health Care*. Belmont: Wadsworth Publishing Company.

Baylis, F., and J. Downie. 1990. *Undergraduate Medical Ethics Education: A Survey of Canadian Medical Schools*. London, Ont.: Westminster Institute for Ethics and Values.

Beauchamp, T.L., and J.F. Childress. 1979. *Principles of Biomedical Ethics*. New York: Oxford University Press.

_____. 1994. *Principles of Biomedical Ethics*, 4th ed. New York: Oxford University Press.

Branswell, H. 1996. Woman's plan to abort one twin sparks uproar. *The Ottawa Citizen*. August 6, A1.

Braude, P.R. 1994. Fertilization in Vitro. In *Principles of Health Care Ethics*, edited by R. Gillon. Chichester: John Wiley & Sons.

Brecher, B. 1994. Organs for Transplants: Donation or Payment? In *Principles of Health Care Ethics*, edited by R. Gillon. Chichester: John Wiley & Sons.

Breckenridge, J., and D. Saunders. 1995. Bitter medicine. *The Globe and Mail*. June 3, D1, D5.

Brett, A.S., and L.B. McCullough. 1986. When patients request specific interventions: Defining the limits of the physician's obligation. *New England Journal of Medicine* 315:1347-1351.

Bricker, E.M. 1989. Industrial marketing and medical ethics. *New England Journal of Medicine* 320:1690-1692.

Brown, K., and A. Jameton. 1993. Commentary. *Hastings Center Report* 23(4):17.

Bruni, F. 1996. Baby's move ends a battle over her fate. *The New York Times*. March 1, B1, B2.

Callahan, D. 1990. Current Trends in Biomedical Ethics in the United States. In *Bioethics: Issues and Perspectives*, edited by S.S. Connor and H.L. Fuenzalida-Puelma. Washington: Pan American Health Organization.

Callahan, D. 1992. Commentary. *Hastings Center Report* 22(1):42.

Campbell, A., G. Gillet, and G. Jones. 1992. *Practical Medical Ethics*. Aukland: Oxford University Press.

Capron, A.M. 1995. Baby Ryan and virtual futility. *Hastings Center Report* 25(2):20-21.

Carrese, J. 1993. Commentary. *Hastings Center Report* 23(4):16.

Chira, S. 1994. New medical quandry at heart of a trial. *The New York Times*. August 3, p.17.

Chrenn, M.M., S. Landefeld, and T.H. Murray. 1989. Doctors, drug companies, and gifts. *Journal of the American Medical Association* 262:3448-3451.

Clement, C.D., and R.C. Sider. 1983. Medical ethics' assault upon medical values. *Journal of the American Medical Association* 250:2011-2015.

Cohen, L. 1989. An ethics committee's ethical dilemma. *Western Report* 4(1):23.

Connor, S.S., and H.L. Fuenzalida-Puelma, eds. 1990. *Bioethics: Issues and Perspectives*. Washington: Pan American Health Organization.

Craig, O. 1997. The right to be grandparents. *The Ottawa Citizen*. October 12, F8.

Ehrenreich, J.D. 1996. Worms, witchcraft and wild incantations: The case of the chicken soup cure. *Anthropological Quarterly* 69(3):137-141.

Eichenwald, E. 1997. Push for royalties threatens use of Down Syndrome test. *The New York Times*. May 23, p.1, D3.

Elliott, J. 1996. Hospital gave placebo for pain, man says. *The Ottawa Citizen*. June 21, C1, C2.

Ellos, E.J. 1990. *Ethical Practice in Clinical Medicine*. London: Routledge.

English, D.C. 1994. *Bioethics: A Clinical Guide for Medical Students*. New York: W.W. Norton & Company.

Evans, M. 1994. Against Brainstem Death. In *Principles of Health Care Ethics*, edited by R. Gillon. Chichester: John Wiley & Sons.

Fins, J.J. 1992. Commentary. *Hastings Center Report* 22(1):41-42.

Fischer, D.S. 1992. Observations on ethical problems and terminal care. *The Yale Journal of Biology and Medicine* 65:105-120.

Fleck, L. 1995. Commentary. *Hastings Center Report* 25(5):29.

Francoeur, R.T. 1983. *Biomedical Ethics: A Guide to Decision Making*. New York: John Wiley & Sons.

Gilligan, C. (1982). *In A Different Voice*. Cambridge, MA: Harvard University Press.

Gillon, R., ed. 1994. Ethical Problems of Scientific Advance—Introduction. *Principles of Health Care Ethics*. Chichester: John Wiley & Sons.

Grant, A. 1993. Questions of life and death. *Canadian Nurse* 89(5):31-34.

Harron, F., J. Burnside, and T. Beauchamp. 1983. *Health and Human Values: A Guide to Making Your Own Decisions*. New Haven: Yale University Press.

Herbert, B. 1994. Profits before patients. *The New York Times*. September 11, 4.19.

_____. 1996. Hidden agenda. *The New York Times*. July 15, A13.

_____. 1996. Torture by H.M.O. *The New York Times*. March 15, A29.

Hodgkinson, C. 1996. *Administrative Philosophy: Values and Motivations in Administrative Life*. Oxford: Pergamon Press.

Jonsen, A.R., and S. Toulmin. 1988. *The Abuse of Casuistry: A History of Moral Reasoning*. Berkeley: University of California Press.

Kantor, J. 1989. *Medical Ethics for Physicians-in-Training*. New York: Plenum Medical Book Company.

Kilborn, P.T. 1997. Doctors organize to fight corporate intrusion. *The New York Times*. July 1, A12.

Kluge, E-H.W. 1992. *Biomedical Ethics in a Canadian Context*. Scarborough: Prentice-Hall Canada, Inc.

Kolata, G. 1994. Battle over a baby's future raises hard ethical issues. *The New York Times*. December 27, A1, A12.

_____. 1995. Withholding care from patients: Boston case asks, who decides? *The New York Times*. April 3, p.1, B8.

Lamb, D. 1994. What is Death. In *Principles of Health Care Ethics*, edited by R. Gillon. Chichester: John Wiley & Sons.

La Puma, J., and D. Schaidermeyer. 1994. *Ethics Consultation: A Practical Guide.* Boston and London: Jones & Bartlett Publishers.

Lavery, J. 1992. When merely staying alive is morally intolerable. *The Globe and Mail.* January 7, A13.

Loewy, E.H. 1989. *Textbook of Medical Ethics.* New York and London: Plenum Medical Book Company.

Lowry, M. 1994. Bad medicine? *Calgary Herald.* September 3, B6.

Macdonald, J.E. and C.L. Beck-Dudley. 1994. Are deontology and teleology mutually exclusive? *Journal of Business Ethics* 13: 615-623.

Malloy, D.C. and H. Hansen. (1995). An holistic model of ethical decision-making for education administration. *Journal of Educational Administration and Foundations* 10(2):60-71.

Marshall, E. 1990. When commerce and academe collide. *Science* 248(4952):152-156

McGinn, C. 1992. *Moral Literacy or How to Do the Right Thing.* London: Gerald Duckworth & Co. Ltd.

McLeod, D. 1991. Drug firms' payola practice under fire. *American Association of Retired Persons Bulletin* 32(2):4.

Medline, E. 1996. Lawyer wants doctor's penalty kept secret. *The Ottawa Citizen.* June 29, C1.

_____. 1996. Medical students believe perks from drug companies acceptable: Half would accept a freebie, study finds. *The Ottawa Citizen.* November 2, A3.

Meyer, M., and T. Weinstein. 1997. A deadly serious fight. *Newsweek.* May 19, p.60.

Miles, S.H. 1990. Why a hospital seeks to discontinue care against family wishes. *Law, Medicine, Health Care* 18:424-425.

_____. 1991. Informed demand for "non-beneficial" medical treatment. *New England Journal of Medicine* 325:512-515.

Mungan, C., and G. Abbate. 1992. Sentence suspended in euthanasia case. *The Globe and Mail.* August 25, A1, A12.

Nicholson, R.H. 1994. The good received, the giver is forgot. *Hastings Center Report* 24(4):5.

Pence, G.E. 1990. *Classic Cases in Medical Ethics: Accounts of the Cases that Have Shaped Medical Ethics, with Philosophical, Legal, and Historical Backgrounds.* New York: McGraw-Hill.

Post, S.G. 1995. Commentary, *Hastings Center Report* 25(5):28.

Rawlins, M.D. 1984. Doctors and the drug makers. *Lancet* ii:276-278.

Rawls, John. 1971. *Theory of Justice.* Cambridge, MA.: Harvard University Press.

Reuters. 1997. Surrogate mother carries twins from separate donors. *The Ottawa Citizen*, March 8, A19.

Rest, J.R. 1984. The major components of morality. In *Morality, Moral Behavior, and Moral Development*, edited by W.M. Kurtines and J.L. Gewrtz (pp. 24-40). New York: John Wiley & Sons.

Sartre, J. 1997. Existentialism. In *Introducing Philosophy: A Text with Integrated Readings*, edited by R.C. Solomon ((pp. 586-589). Toronto, ON: Harcourt Brace College Publishers.

Sass, H-M. 1990. Bioethics: Its Philosophical Bases and Application. In *Bioethics: Issues and Perspectives*, edited by S.S. Connor and H.L. Fuenzaleda-Puelma. Washington, D.C.: Pan American Health Organization.

Sells, R.A. 1994. Transplants. In *Principles of Health Care Ethics*, edited by R. Gillon. Chichester: John Wiley & Sons.

Sergeant, M.D., P.G. Hodgetts, M. Godwin, D.M.C. Walker, and P. McHenry. 1996. Interactions with the pharmaceutical industry: A survey of family medicine residents in Ontario. *Canadian Medical Association Journal* 155(9):1243-1248.

Shea, E.J. 1996. *Ethical Decisions in Sport: Interscholastic, Intercollegiate, Olympic and Professional*. Springfield: Charles C. Thomas, Publishers.

Shimm, D.S., and R.G. Spence. 1991. Industry reimbursement for entering patients into clinical trials: Legal and ethical issues. *Annals of Internal Medicine* 115(2):148-151.

Siegal, B. 1997. Waiting for a miracle. *The Ottawa Citizen*. February 15, B1, B4.

Snowden, R., and E. Snowden. 1994. Ethical Problems in Infertility Treatment. In *Principles of Health Care Ethic*, edited by R. Gillon. Chichester: John Wiley & Sons.

Trevino, L.K. 1986. Ethical decision making in organizations: A person-interactionist model. *Academy of Management Review* 11:601-617.

U.S. Department of Health and Human Services. 1996. Physical Activity and Health: A Report of the Surgeon General. Atlanta, Ga.: U.S. Department of Health and Human Services, Centers for Disease Control and Prevention, National Center for Chronic Disease Prevention and Health Promotion.

Van De Veer, H., and T. Regan, eds. 1987. *Health Care Ethics. An Introduction*. Philadelphia: Temple University Press.

Veatch, R.M. 1977. *Case Studies in Medical Ethics*. Cambridge: Harvard University Press.

Walker, R. 1994. Alberta college investigating six MDs for practicing chelation therapy. *Medical Post*. October 25, 12.

_____. 1995. Alternative therapies may soon get nod. *Calgary Herald*. October 6, A4.

Wall, T.F. 1980. *Medical Ethics: Basic Moral Issues*. Washington: University Press of America, Inc.

Weaver, M. 1996. Woman carrying eight fetuses risks health of self and babies. *The Ottawa Citizen*. August 10, A10.

Weston, B., and M. Lauria. 1996. Patient advocacy in the 1990s. *New England Journal of Medicine* 334(8):543-544.

Williams, J.R. 1986. *Biomedical Ethics in Canada*. Lewston/Queenston: The Edwin Mellon Press.

Witt, M.D., and L.O. Gosten. 1994. Conflict of interest dilemmas in biomedical research. *Journal of the American Medical Association* 271(7):547-551.

Unauthored articles:

[No Author]. 1992. What judge said of woman's right to die. *The Toronto Star*. January 8, A12.

[No Author]. 1992. Palliation in the age of chronic disease. *Hastings Center Report* 22(1):41.

[No Author]. 1993. Culture, healing, and professional obligations. *Hastings Center Report* 23(4):15.

[No Author]. 1994. Ethics issue over doctor as legal consultant. *The New York Times*. December 13, B10.

[No Author]. 1995. My conscience, your money. *Hastings Center Report* 25(5):28.

[No Author]. 1996. Potential mother of 8 to be paid per live baby. *The Ottawa Citizen*. August 12, A6.

[No Author]. 1996. Octuplet mother pledges to have all her babies. *The Ottawa Citizen*. August 11, A2.

[No Author]. 1996. Woman pregnant with 8 rejects abortion advice. *The Toronto Star*. August 11, A5.

Index